AIDS and alcohol/drug abuse

"There is some fascinating and troubling reading in this collection [of chapters] that highlights the devastating effect of AIDS and intravenous drug use among minority populations. I feel this volume will benefit clinician researchers and will be of great interest to public policy officials. The ethical issues faced in this major public health problem are straightforwardly addressed and are nicely summarized."

Yvonne Connelly, MA, Quality Assurance Coordinator, Department of Psychiatry, Duke University Medical Center, Durham, North Carolina

AIDS and
Alcohol/Drug Abuse:
Psychosocial Research

ISBN 0-918393-85-X

Published by

Harrington Park Press, 10 Alice Street, Binghamton, NY 13904-1580
EUROSPAN/Harrington, 3 Henrietta Street, London WC2E 8LU England

Harrington Park Press is a subsidiary of The Haworth Press, Inc., 10 Alice Street, Binghamton, NY 13904-1580.

AIDS and Alcohol/Drug Abuse: Psychosocial Research was originally published as *Drugs & Society*, Volume 5, Numbers 1/2 1990.

Cover design by Marshall Andrews.

Library of Congress Cataloging-in-Publication Data

AIDS and alcohol/drug abuse : psychosocial research / Dennis G. Fisher, editor.
    p. cm.
    "Simultaneously issued by The Haworth Press, Inc., under the same title, as a special issue of Drugs & society, volume 5, numbers 1/2, 1990"
    Includes bibliographical references.
    ISBN 0-918393-85-X (pbk. : alk. paper)
    1. AIDS (Disease) — Social aspects. 2. Substance abuse — Social aspects. 3. AIDS (Disease) — Psychological aspects. 4. Substance abuse — Psychological aspects. I. Fisher, Dennis G.
    [DNLM: 1. Acquired Immunodeficiency Syndrome. 2. Alcoholism. 3. Minority Groups. 4. Psychology, Social. 5. Research — methods. 6. Substance Abuse, Intravenous. WD 308 A28772]
RA644.A25A3323 1990
616.97'92071 — dc20
DNLM/DLC
for Library of Congress

90-5312
CIP

AIDS and
Alcohol/Drug Abuse:
Psychosocial Research

Dennis G. Fisher, PhD
Editor

AIDS and Alcohol/Drug Abuse: Psychosocial Research was simultaneously issued by The Haworth Press, Inc., under the same title, as a special issue of *Drugs & Society*, Volume 5, Numbers 1/2 1990, Dennis G. Fisher, Editor.

The Harrington Park Press
New York • London

Dedication

This volume is dedicated to the memory of Paul Devore and others like him who have succumbed to the ravages of this plague of AIDS.

Royalties from the sale of this publication will be donated to:

AIDS Hospice Foundation
Paul Devore's Fund
1800 North Argyle Avenue, Suite 304
Los Angeles, California 90028
(213) 462-2273

CONTENTS

ABOUT THE EDITOR

Dennis G. Fisher, PhD, is Assistant Professor in the Center for Alcohol and Addiction Studies at the University of Alaska-Anchorage. He was a National Institute on Drug Abuse Epidemiology Fellow in Quantitative Psychology at the University of California, Los Angeles. The first field representative for the Drug Abuse Division of the Joint Commission on Accreditation of Hospitals, Dr. Fisher was also the previous program evaluation supervisor for the Bureau of Drug Abuse of the State of Ohio.

Preface

The immediacy of AIDS was personally brought home to me by the death of my brother Paul Devore. It is only fitting that this volume contains a most unique collection of papers about the deadly disease that claimed Paul's life among many others, as Paul was a most unique individual. AIDS is the number one health issue facing the nation today. How AIDS relates to substance abuse is the theme of this volume. The papers are concerned with aspects of HIV infection that have not received very much attention elsewhere.

The article by Des Jarlais, Casriel, Stepherson, and Friedman, sets the stage for several of the papers that follow by pointing out the problems of doing AIDS research on racial minorities in this country. That disease has had such devastating effect on racial minorities that there is a danger of additional stigmatization of those communities. The pitfalls that have befallen some researchers are poignantly illustrated by this powerful discussion. Anyone doing research on AIDS involving ethnic minorities should seriously consider the points raised by this paper.

The next article by Fisher, Wilson, and Brause, is the first paper about intravenous drug use in Alaska ever published in the open literature. The paper is mostly descriptive because that is the place to start i.e., by describing and documenting what is already known but what has never been made available to the scientific community. It is important to start documenting what has been taking place because of a prediction of a devastating epidemic of HIV infection among Alaska Natives.

A warning to start paying attention to both American Indians and Alaskan Natives is presented by Ron Rowell who is the director of the National Native American AIDS Prevention Center. Rowell

xiii

himself is a full-blooded Choctaw/Kaskaskia Indian. He presents some little-known facts that relate substance abuse to HIV infection in the American Indian/Alaskan Native population.

Problems with prevention, research, and treatment of individuals who are both intravenous drug users and who are infected with HIV are discussed by Dennis Leoutsakas. Dennis is a board member of the National Association of People With Aids (NAPWA), one of the founders and the president of the Board of Trustees of Alaskans Living with HIV (ALHIV), and one of the founders and a board member of the World HIV network. His insight into the practical, policy, and ethical issues involved in this complex topic will be appreciated by those struggling with this population themselves.

Martin and Hasin present an analysis of data from 604 gay men in New York City. The data concern alcohol and sexual behavior. These data demonstrate that there have been important changes in sexual behavior by gay men especially in relation to alcohol use. However, there is still a major problem with gay men who are alcoholics. We need this important information about the interaction between alcohol consumption and high-risk sexual behavior because alcohol is the number one drug of abuse.

One of the most powerful ethnographic studies ever written is presented by Page, Smith, and Kane who describe in chilling detail the actual process of transmission of HIV in shooting galleries in Miami, Florida. Anyone doing work in the field of AIDS prevention will be mesmerized by this paper which tells the stories of people essentially infecting themselves with HIV (or putting themselves at extreme risk of HIV) and presents those stories from the standpoint of the researcher who was present while it was going on.

The paper by James Sorensen has been selected to be last in this sequence because, like the last being to be let out of Pandora's box, Sorensen presents hope. There is hope for intravenous drug users and AIDS prevention. Sorensen suggests that the basis for AIDS prevention work with intravenous drug users is based on models of health psychology although they do not fit perfectly. The "Bleach Man" approach that Sorensen describes is well-known to AIDS prevention workers and his paper is truly an upbeat delight.

Dennis G. Fisher, PhD

Expectations of Racial Prejudice in AIDS Research and Prevention Programs in the United States

Don C. Des Jarlais, PhD
Cathy Casriel, CSW
Bruce Stepherson, BA
Samuel R. Friedman, PhD

SUMMARY. HIV infection and AIDS have occurred at disproportionately higher rates among Black and Hispanic persons in the United States. The HIV epidemic is occurring within an historical context of racial prejudice and inequality within the society as a whole, and of poor health care for minority communities. We report instances of expectations of racial prejudice that affected three different AIDS research/prevention activities. Failure to anticipate and appropriately respond to these expectations of racial prejudice may substantially interfere with AIDS efforts and appear to confirm the expectations. Even with the best anticipation and responses, there will be many instances in which the problem cannot be satisfactorily resolved. The association of AIDS with minority status has the potential to reinforce stigmatization of minority communities. Prevention and research activities will often be caught in lose-lose situations of either "unfairly singing out" minorities or of ignoring the problems of minority communities.

The AIDS epidemic is having a disproportionate impact on minority communities in the United States. As of April 29, 1989, 27% of the AIDS cases reported to the Centers for Disease Control have

Don C. Des Jarlais is affiliated with The Beth Israel Medical Center, 1st Avenue and 16th Street, New York, NY 10003.

Cathy Casriel, Bruce Stepherson, and Samuel R. Friedman are affiliated with The Narcotic and Drug Research, Inc., 11 Beach Street, New York, NY 10013.

occurred in Black (African) Americans and 15% in Latino (Hispanic) Americans (Centers for Disease Control, 1989). These percentages are more than double the percentages of Blacks (12%) and Latinos (6%) in the U.S. population as a whole (U.S. Bureau of the Census, 1981). Much (but not all) of this overrepresentation is due to Blacks and Latinos who were exposed to HIV through the sharing of equipment for injecting illicit drugs, and also to heterosexual and perinatal transmission from those drug injectors. Blacks comprise 51% and Latinos 29% of the cases in which drug injection is the primary risk behavior.

Even among intravenous drug users, there are indications of higher risk for HIV infection and AIDS for Blacks and Latinos in the United States. Various studies have found significant differences in HIV seroprevalence rates among IV drug users by ethnic group (see the review by Hahn, Onorato, Jones, & Dougherty, 1989). In several of these studies the ethnic group differences did not remain statistically significant after controlling for drug use behavior (e.g., in Marmor et al. 1987; Weiss et al. 1987), but in all of the studies, the direction of the ethnic differences was for higher rates in ethnic minorities compared to White intravenous drug users. The reason(s) for these differences are not yet understood.

The disproportionate number of AIDS cases among Blacks and Latinos, and the higher seroprevalence rates among ethnic minority IV drug users, argue strongly for both more research to explain the differences and for immediate AIDS prevention efforts focussed on minority group members at risk for HIV infection. It would be a fundamental mistake, however, to assume that such research and prevention efforts will automatically be seen as good faith attempts to understand and limit the spread of HIV. Instead, many research and prevention programs are likely to be seen as extensions of a previous history of inadequate health care provided to minority communities, including ethnic prejudice on the part of some authorities. There is certainly sufficient historical evidence for adopting such a perspective (Willis, 1987).

Expectations of racial prejudice can both prevent needed research and reduce participation in AIDS prevention programs. This paper presents three such instances in which the authors were involved. While different choices by the researchers might have reduced the extent to which the expectations of racial prejudice were activated, in all three of these instances the very nature of the intervention or research project triggered the expectations. Failure to try the intervention or collect the data would also have been seen as racist, however, in that it could be construed as ignoring the problem of HIV infection in minority communities.

As part of the Centers for Disease Control "Innovative AIDS Prevention Studies" program, we have been conducting a study on the transition from non-injecting to injecting drug use. Appropriate subjects for the study were persons who were currently sniffing, but not injecting, heroin. Recruitment was done through asking known sniffers to refer their friends and acquaintances, having street workers hand out cards, and placing advertisements in New York City newspapers. The cards and the newspaper advertisements stated "Heroin Sniffers. Research Study Needs You for Paid Interviews. Call (phone number)."

When potential subjects called, they were asked a brief set of questions on demographics and drug use. The eligibility criteria were that a subject in the full study had to have sniffed heroin in the last 6 months, could not be currently injecting drugs, and was 18 or older. Subjects who met these criteria were then asked to come in for a longer face-to-face interview and blood sample for which they would be paid $20. We did not tell the potential subjects what the criteria were because we did not want to tempt them to give false information just so that they could participate in the study and gain the $20. These telephone screening interviews were conducted by both White and Black interviewers.

In order to better understand who was being reached through the recruitment process, we asked about demographic characteristics and about how subjects had heard of the study as part of the telephone screening interview. With both our White and Black interviewers, potential subjects were often hesitant to answer the ethnicity question. Eventually one potential subject, whose history of intensive heroin injection disqualified him for the study, directly accused us of racial prejudice. When told that he would not be included in the full study, he stated "It's because I'm Black isn't it. You took my friend who is White and you're not taking me because I'm Black."

Following this incident, we deleted the ethnicity question on the screening interview. This did not, however, allay all suspicions of racial prejudice. Both Black and White interviewers continued to note intimations that ineligible subjects believed their ethnicity was a basis for disqualification. (Subjects probably believed that naming specific community newspapers in answer to the question "How did you hear about the study?" revealed their ethnicity.)

Face-to-face contact between eligible subjects and project staff usually alleviated suspicions about prejudice and the project as a whole. During the face-to-face interviews, we were often told "You look like a nice person" or "I know I can trust you." These judgments were made on a basis of a personal appraisal of the interviewer, rather than on any institutional affiliation.

In this study, expectations of racial prejudice clearly reduced our ability to collect data on potential participants. Because potential subjects were asked to refer other heroin sniffers, the expectations of prejudice almost certainly kept some additional persons from participation.

Expectations of racial prejudice in AIDS research and prevention programs do not only occur at the level of the individual. They also occur at the community level and affect the political processes involved in AIDS research and prevention programs. Under contract with the Centers for Disease Control, the Research Triangle Institute had planned to conduct a pilot study for a national HIV sero-prevalence study.[1] This pilot study was to be conducted in Washington, DC, primarily because RTI had a field office in Washington, and the AIDS case rate in Washington indicated that there should be a high enough seroprevalence rate to justify pilot testing. The pilot study included experimental variation: randomly selected subjects were to be offered payment to determine if this would increase the participation rate. Communication between RTI, several Black AIDS service organizations and the District Health Department about the study did occur prior to the planned starting date of the pilot test. This communication, however, was not sufficient for the Commissioner of Health to feel fully apprised of the study, nor for accurate information about the nature of the study to disseminate

---

[1] DCD is a member of the National Advisory Board for this pilot study.

through the informal networks within the Black community. The lack of adequate communication undoubtedly contributed to the later negative public response. Just prior to the beginning of field interviewing, the Washington media gave intensive coverage to the study, including an analogy to the Tuskegee syphilis study. (This analogy was made by a Black community leader who had not been included in the earlier meetings.) Because of the community response, the pilot test for Washington was cancelled. A pilot test has since been implemented in the Pittsburgh/Allegheny County area, with greater prior involvement of the political leadership of the Black community.

In New York City, syringe exchange programs to reduce the spread of HIV among intravenous drug users have been discussed since 1985.[2] Final approvals for a limited pilot study were obtained by the City Department of Health in August, 1988. One of the explicit objections to the pilot study was that such a study would be "racist" because most of the participants in the study would likely be minority drug users (Joseph, 1988). The pilot syringe exchange is currently operational in New York, but community pressure has limited the number of sites, and thus the number of potential participants.[3]

As noted above, there is sufficient historical justification for expectations of prejudice/racism towards minority group members in the United States, particularly with respect to health care. These expectations exist at both an individual level and a community/public action level. Ignorance of or insensitivity to these expectations by researchers and public health officials can easily lead to problematic interactions, delays in implementation of AIDS prevention activities, and apparent confirmation of the original expectations.

It is important also to note the double bind nature of some of the expectations of racial prejudice. If high percentages of minority group members are to participate in the study or prevention program, then a charge of racism can be made on a basis of the program appearing to "unfairly single out" minorities. If few minority

---

[2]Authors DCD and SRF have both participated in these discussions.
[3]Due to the election of a new mayor the New York City syringe exchange program has been closed.

group members are to participate in the study, then the charge of racism can be made on the basis of using race to exclude, or on a basis of not meeting the needs of minority communities.

A double bind also exists from the perspective of minority communities. Findings of a high prevalence of AIDS related problems in minority communities can be used to further stigmatize those communities, while findings of a low prevalence of AIDS related problems can be used to justify not allocating public resources for the problems.

We do not want to leave the impression that nothing can or should be done to address the spread of HIV in ethnic minority communities in the United States. There are a variety of ways of reducing expectations of racial prejudice in AIDS research and prevention activities. These include having minority group members in positions of leadership and having face-to-face contact between researchers, service providers and participants. It is important that researchers listen carefully to community concerns and modify the programs and studies before implementation. We want to emphasize that current AIDS prevention activities will have to anticipate and work with expectations of racial prejudice. In many ways, the situation is best summarized by a quotation from Beny Primm of the Presidential Commission on the HIV Epidemic: "If you do something now, you will be accused of racism, but if you do nothing now, in the future you will be accused of genocide." (B. Primm, Personal communication during discussions at First AIDS and Minorities Conference in Atlanta, April, 1987. Used with permission).

REFERENCES

Centers for Disease Control (1989, April). *HIV/AIDS Surveillance*.U.S. Bureau of the Census (1981). *1980 Census of the population, characteristics of the population*, 1. Washington: United States Department of Commerce.

Hahn, R. A., Onorato, I. M., Jones, T. S., & Dougherty, J. (1989). The prevalence of infection with Human Immunodeficiency Virus among intravenous drug users in the U.S. *Journal of the American Medical Association, 261*(18), 2677-2684.

Joseph, S. (1988, October 18). *Current challenges of aids in New York City*. Paper presented at Montefiore Annual AIDS Conference, New York,.

Marmor, M., Des Jarlais, D. C., Cohen, H., Friedman, S. R., Beatrice, S. T., Dubin, N., El-Sadr, W., Mildvan, D., Yancovitz, S., Mathur, U., & Holtzman, R. (1987). Risk factors for Infection with Human Immunodeficiency Virus among intravenous drug abusers in New York City. *AIDS*, *1*, 39-44.

Weiss, S. H., Ginzburg, H. M., Goedert, J. J., Biggar, R. J., Blattner, W.A. et al. (1985, April). Risk for HTLV-III exposure and AIDS among parenteral drug abusers in New Jersey. Paper presented at the International Conference on the Acquired Immunodeficiency Syndrome (AIDS), Atlanta, Georgia.

Willis, D. P. (Ed.) (1987). Currents of health policy: Impacts on Black Americans. *Milbank Quarterly*, *65* (suppl 1 & 2).

Intravenous Drug Use in Alaska

Dennis G. Fisher, PhD
Patricia J. Wilson, PHN, BS
Jay Brause

SUMMARY. This paper is the first report specifically devoted to intravenous drug use (IVDU) in Alaska to appear in the open literature. Primary or secondary analysis of existing data sources was performed to accomplish this focus. The data sources were: the statewide survey of drug use in the public schools (Segal, 1988), a study of clients in treatment in substance abuse programs (Fisher & Brause, 1988), an unpublished survey of IVDUs by outreach workers at an AIDS prevention program (Johnson & Wilson, 1988), a snowball survey of gays and lesbians in Alaska (Identity, Incorporated, 1986), and a household survey of adults in Fairbanks (Booker & Hellekson, 1988, November). The conclusions are that Alaska has a major problem with intravenous drug use and that intravenous drug users are a potential vector of Human Immunodeficiency Virus (HIV) infection to the non-IVDU population within the state.

There have been no publications in the open literature which have dealt specifically with intravenous drug use in Alaska. This paper is a first. As a consequence of the lack of information on the topic, many drug researchers are under the misimpression that there is no drug use — certainly no intravenous drug use — in Alaska. Nothing could be further from the truth. Alaska has consistently had one of the highest if not the highest rate of alcoholism and alcohol use of any state in the nation. Per capita, Alaska spends more money on

Dennis G. Fisher, Patricia J. Wilson and Jay Brause are affiliated with the Center for Alcohol and Addiction Studies, University of Alaska-Anchorage.

Correspondence should be addressed to Dennis G. Fisher, Center for Alcohol and Addiction Studies, University of Alaska-Anchorage, 3211 Providence Drive, Anchorage, AK 99508.

narcotics law enforcement than any state in the nation (E. Harter, personal communication). The statewide surveys of substance use in the public schools have also demonstrated consistently high use of substances as compared to other states and national surveys (Segal, 1988; Segal, McKelvy, Bowman, & Mala, 1983, July 31).

This paper will both review several technical reports and heretofore unpublished data that describe intravenous (IV) drug use in Alaska. The reports are being cited as the source of data, but the data in all cases are reanalyzed for this publication to focus on intravenous use.

DESCRIPTION OF REPORTS

Statewide Survey of Public School Students

Segal (1988) surveyed 4,129 public school students in grades 7-12 in eight school districts. Six school districts had been originally surveyed in 1983: Anchorage, Barrow, Bethel, Fairbanks, Juneau, Kotzebue, Nome, and Sitka. Two others were added in 1988. They were Cordova and Seward. In some cases a stratified random sample of the school population was performed. In other cases the appropriate grade levels of the entire school were surveyed. Segal was able to collect information about intravenous cocaine use and heroin use. Segal states, "Alaska's prevalence levels, except for lifetime experience with alcohol and depressants among high school seniors, exceeded those reported in national surveys. Moreover, Alaska's lifetime prevalence levels generally exceed or match results from California or Oregon for comparably matched students" (p. 18).

Segal's data includes questions on the use of heroin and the intravenous use of cocaine. The route of administration was not collected for the heroin use. It is possible that the heroin may have been smoked or snorted. For the purposes of this paper we will assume that the heroin was injected. This is quite plausible as all of the heroin reported by outreach workers in 1988 was of a type that is reportedly very difficult to smoke or snort. The Alaska State Troopers (AST) corroborate the report of the outreach workers in that all heroin seized by the AST was what the AST call Mexican

Brown or black tar heroin. Mexican heroin comes into Alaska through Seattle (Alaska State Troopers [AST], 1989, p. 13). They also report that in 1988 all reports were of injection and no reports of snorting or smoking (D. Bowman, personal communication, March 23, 1989). We will also equate needle use with intravenous injection although it is possible that intramuscular injection was performed.

There were 89 individuals who reported use of either one of these drugs. Seventy reported use of heroin, 23 reported intravenous use of cocaine. As Schwarcz and Rutherford (1989) have pointed out, a major vector of HIV transmission for adolescents can well be through shared needles in intravenous drug use. Sixteen of the 89 reported use of both drugs which meant that only 7 respondents intravenously used cocaine without using heroin. Whites were the majority of users of either drug, with Alaskan Natives making up the second largest group. This was partially due to the larger numbers of Whites and Alaskan Natives in the overall sample as it was the proportion of Hispanics within the overall sample who were IVDUs which was significantly higher than the proportion of Alaskan Natives ($z = 2.96, p < .01$), Whites ($z = 2.41, p < .05$), and Other ($z = 1.99$, p $< .05$). No significant sex differences in overall use of either drug were detected. However there was a significant difference in the age of first use of cocaine with girls ($M = 12.5$) starting use of cocaine before boys ($M = 13.7$), $t(68) = 2.44$, $p = .0169$. This may be because girls are more easily able to obtain cocaine by trading sex for the drug. (Data relevant to this question are reported in the Outreach Worker Contact section of this paper.) The link between cocaine and sexual activity has been reported by others (Center for Disease Control [CDC], 1989, March 17). There were no significant differences in the age of first use of heroin. There were large correlations between age of first use of heroin and age of first use of cocaine for both those who only injected one drug ($r = .67, p = .0001$) and those who injected both drugs ($r = .56$, p $= .0316$). The mean age of first use of heroin is 13.27 years and the mean age of first use of cocaine (whether injected or not) for this sample is 13.15 years ($n = 70$).

Of those who injected both drugs, the majority were White (60%). Alaskan Natives also made up a large proportion (27%).

There is an impression that IV drug use in Alaska is found primarily in Anchorage and Fairbanks (Tower, 1987, p. 2). Contrary to this impression, only 61% of this sample were from Anchorage or Fairbanks, and only 10% from Juneau. This leaves 29% of the IVDUs in this sample outside the three major population centers of Alaska.

Homosexual, Lesbian, and Bisexual Adults

Identity, Incorporated (1986) distributed 1518 questionnaires to gay, lesbian, and bisexual men and women in Alaska and achieved a return rate of 48% or 734 verified and completed questionnaires. Another 12 questionnaires came back after the report had gone to press. This population had never before been assessed in Alaskan history.

The questionnaire inquired about substance abuse history including intravenous drug use, as well as general demographics, health, and social issues. The mean time in Alaska for the total sample was 9.8 years and over 23% had participated in substance abuse treatment. Over 66% use drugs other than alcohol and 42% use drugs other than marijuana or nitrites. Mean age of the total sample was 31.8 years. Two-thirds were from the Municipality of Anchorage, 19% were from Fairbanks North Star Borough, 9% from the City and Borough of Juneau and 9% other, with 24 cities, towns, and villages represented in total.

Stall and Ostrow (1989, p. 66) have indicated that homosexual men who use needles have seroprevalence rates which approach saturation. It therefore is important for us to examine whatever data are available to us about this group. There were 11 respondents in the Identity, Incorporated (1986) data set who indicated that they used drugs intravenously. All 11 lived in Alaska. There were 1 Hispanic woman, 3 White women, 1 Black man, 2 Hispanic men, and 4 White men. Ages ranged from 24 to 50 with a female mean of 27.5 and a male mean of 34. Three of the women self-identified as lesbian and one as bisexual. All the men self-identified as gay or primarily gay. One man was divorced and all the rest of the sample were single. The men had had 0-6 male sex partners within the last month and 3-50 within the last year ($M = 15$). None of the men had had any female sex partners in the last year. The women had had 1-

10 female sex partners in the last year (M = 4.25). One of the women had had a male sex partner in the last year. All the sample were at least high school graduates with 8 of the sample having at least some college. One man had been in the Army, one in the Navy, and one in the Coast Guard.

All the men were either employed full time or self-employed. Two of the women were employed full time and 2 were not employed. The men (M = $34,600) had significantly greater annual income than the women (M = $8,500), $t(9)$ = 3.35, p = .0085. None of the sample report having any problem with insurance companies due to their sexual orientation.

The sample seemed to have quite a bit of problems with alcohol. Only one man and one woman do not drink alcohol currently. One man usually has 11-15 drinks at a time and two of the women have 6-10 drinks at a time. One woman drinks daily, one man and one woman drink 3-6 times per week. Two woman and 3 men report that their drinking causes depression. The women were significantly more likely to report that drinking cause blackouts (likelihood ratio $\chi^2(1, N = 11)$ = 6.782, p = .009). Three women and 2 men had been arrested for driving while intoxicated. One woman had been counselled for alcohol abuse and had been to treatment for her own alcohol problem.

Drug use patterns have been a major area of concern in the research literature (Stall & Wiley, 1988). This sample had extensive polydrug use. Only one man did not use marijuana or cocaine. All the rest of the sample used both marijuana and cocaine. One woman did not use nitrites. Our data corroborate a relationship reported by Centers for Disease Control Task Force on Kaposi's Sarcoma and Opportunistic Infections (1982) in that there was a significant correlation between frequency of nitrite use and the number of male sexual partners in the past year (r = .699, p = .0166). This may have implications for the development of Kaposi's Sarcoma should any of these individuals become HIV positive (Haverkos, 1988; Haverkos, Pinsky, Drotman, & Bregman, 1985). One woman and 4 men did not use depressants. The women were significantly more likely to report worse general health than the men (likelihood ratio $\chi^2(1, N = 11)$ = 11.648, p = .003). The men in general were significantly more concerned that their lifestyle had personally exposed them to AIDS infection (likelihood ratio $\chi^2(1, N = 11) = 6.782, p = .009$). In fact none of the women were concerned about exposure to AIDS even though all the women used drugs intravenously, 3 used nitrites, and one of the women had had sex with a man within the past year. Concern about this lack of awareness of the risk of HIV infection among lesbian IVDUs has been expressed by Dicker (1989). One of the men who was not concerned about exposure to AIDS had had 15 male sex partners within the past year and used drugs intravenously.

Treatment Program Clients

Fisher and Brause (1988) interviewed 80 clients who were participating in substance abuse treatment in the Municipality of Anchorage. Interview scheduling was attempted with 112 total possible clients but because of program refusals and scheduling errors only 80 were completed for a completion rate of 71%. The mean age was 31.75 years. There were 53 men and 27 women, of whom 3 were Black, 5 were Hispanic, 18 were Alaskan Native, and 54 were White. There were no Black women. The men in treatment were significantly older than the women. Clients had been in treatment a mean of 11 months. Mean number of previous treatment episodes was 2.5. The number of drugs the clients had taken ranged from 0 to 7 with a mean of 2.7.

There were 16 individuals in this data set who used some drug intravenously. There was 1 Black man, 1 Hispanic woman, 2 Alaska Native men, 1 Alaska Native woman, 6 White men, and 5 White women. Eight used cocaine, 5 used heroin, and 4 used amphetamine. One of these drug users used more than one drug intravenously. Eleven of these 16 had been tested for HIV. The 16 IVDUs had about the same mean age as the entire sample – 31.3 – and the men were not significantly older than the women. The IVDUs took slightly more drugs than the sample as a whole for an average of 3.5. All the heroin users were White. There were 3 White and 1 Native amphetamine users. There were 4 White, 2 Native, 1 Hispanic, and 1 Black users of intravenous cocaine. It is noteworthy that none of the Alaska Native IVDUs used heroin. The men were significantly less likely to use heroin than the women (likelihood ratio $\chi^2(1, N = 16) = 4.035, p = .045$). The 16 clients had been in treatment a mean length of 10 months. The mean number of previous treatment episodes was 2.1.

Outreach Worker Contacts

Johnson and Wilson (1988) directed the distribution of 50 questionnaires to intravenous drug users. The questionnaires were distributed by outreach workers at an AIDS prevention program for needle users. Thirty-nine of the questionnaires were completed and returned for a return rate of 78%. The mean age is 33 years and the mean highest grade in school completed is 11. There were 19 female and 20 male drug users. Twenty-one were White, 11 Black, 4 Hispanic, and 3 Alaskan Native. The mean age of first needle use is 21 with a range from 13 to 37. There is a significant correlation between last school grade completed and age of first needle use ($r = .37, p < .05$).

Twenty-three of the sample reported cleaning their needles with bleach, however this may not be effective for infection control as there was significantly more cleaning of works after injection as opposed to before injection ($z = 2.8, p < .01$). Newmeyer, Feldman, Biernacki, and Watters (1989, p. 169) report that new needles in San Francisco could be obtained for about $2. Our IVDUs report that they obtain new needles for a mean of $3.84 ($SD = 2.20).

Of those who injected cocaine the mean number of times injected in the last 30 days prior to the survey is 56 ($n = 22$). An interesting finding about the cocaine users is that there is a negative correlation between number of times injected cocaine and the highest grade in school completed ($r = -.56, p = .0066$), the more education someone had, the less cocaine they used. Of those who injected heroin, the mean number of times injected in the last 30 days is 74 ($n = 24$), and for Dilaudid it is 78 ($n = 22$). There is a strong correlation between the number of times a respondent injected Dilaudid with the number of times a respondent injected heroin for those ($n = 16$) who used both drugs ($r = .97, p = .0001$). There is a slightly weaker correlation between the number of times respondents injected cocaine with the number of times they injected heroin for those ($n = 10$) who used both of these drugs ($r = .91, p =$

.0003). However, there is a very low correlation between cocaine and Dilaudid for those ($n = 7$) who used these two drugs ($r = .05$, NS). This leads us to hypothesize that there are two different groups of intravenous drug users in Anchorage. One group uses heroin and Dilaudid, and the other group uses heroin and cocaine. Controlling for heroin use, a contingency table shows a definite separation between Dilaudid use and cocaine use (Fisher exact $p = .032$). Of the 3 Alaskan Natives in this study 2 used both heroin and Dilaudid, while one used only Dilaudid. This contrasts with the Fisher and Brause (1988) study in which none of the Native IVDUs used opiates. This raises the question of treatment accessibility for Alaskan Native IVDU opiate users.

One of the concerns that prompted Johnson and Wilson to conduct their study is the potential for these intravenous drug users to be vectors of AIDS transmission to the non-intravenous-drug-using population. Their fears may be justified as 58% of this sample had sex with non-users in the 30 days prior to the survey and only 32% used condoms. Women were much more likely to have sex in order to obtain drugs, adj. $\chi^2(1, N = 39) = 10.44$, $p < .001$. The difficulty with getting men to use condoms has been pointed out in the literature (Solomon & DeJong, 1989; Valdiserri, Arena, Proctor, & Bonati, 1989). Our data corroborate this as women were also more likely to use condoms, adj. $\chi^2(1, N = 38) = 3.87$, $p < .05$. These data suggest the extent of prostitution among female intravenous drug users and the fact that the prostitutes are protecting themselves against infection through the use of condoms.

Household Survey of Adults in Fairbanks

Three hundred ten randomly selected adult (21 years or older) residents of the Fairbanks North Star Borough were interviewed for one hour each. The residents were interviewed as part of a study of Seasonal Affective Disorder (Booker & Hellekson, 1988, November). The overall sample was 50% women, 6% Alaska Native, and 9% Black. The median age is 37 years, 12% were born in Alaska, and 50% had been in Alaska for 13 years or longer. Ninety-five percent had at least a high school education, and 21% had college or professional degrees. There were 29 residents who had taken opioids in the past year without a prescription. Analysis of data concerning this sample of 29 opioid users is presented here.

The mean age of this sample is 34.7 years. The men and the women are not significantly different in age. There are 15 White men, and 9 White women, 3 Black women, 1 Oriental woman, and 1 Alaska Native/American Indian woman. Fourteen of these people had some college or vocational school; 8 graduated high school or GED; 4 had BA/BS degrees; 1 had less than high school; 1 had a doctorate; 1 was listed as other. The men smoked more cigarettes ($M = 67.4$) than the women ($M = 37.9$) but not significantly so. The interesting finding from these data is that the women were more likely to use drugs other than opioids than the men ($\chi^2(1, N = 29) = 4.243, p = .039$). The drugs the women were using were marijuana, cocaine, and amphetamine. None of the men used amphetamines and only one used cocaine, whereas 3 of the women used amphetamine and 3 used cocaine. Even though the numbers are small, this finding is consistent with other findings presented in this paper.

DISCUSSION

This paper presents results from all known datasets concerning intravenous drug use in Alaska or datasets from which information could reasonably be extracted that bears on intravenous drug use in Alaska. A major point that is supported by several of the datasets is that female IVDUs seem to be particularly attracted to stimulants, especially cocaine and amphetamine. An impressive finding in this regard is the mean age of first cocaine use for female intravenous drug users of 12.5 years. This would imply that these adolescent girls may be at particular risk for blood-borne infections such as hepatitis-B and HIV. It may also imply that adolescent female IV-DUs may be at risk for sexually transmitted diseases if they are exchanging sex for drugs such as cocaine. Even though the older female IVDUs are reporting use of condoms in their sexual activity, it is doubtful whether the younger female IVDUs are using condoms. Howard, Stovall, and Farrell (1989, August) report that only a small number of 7th graders used any kind of contraception compared to a much larger number who engaged in sexual intercourse.

The possibility of needle-sharing must also be raised as it is questionable whether 12.5 year old girls are concerned enough to practice good hygiene in their injection techniques. We predict that intravenous drug use and unprotected sex with multiple sex partners is going to be a double vector of HIV infection into the adolescent population and that at least a segment of the adolescent population will show high seroprevalence levels in the near future.

Another issue that needs to be dealt with through prevention education is the feeling among lesbian and bisexual female IVDUs that their homosexual activity makes them somehow immune to HIV infection even though they use drugs intravenously and have sex with men. The striking correlation between the use of nitrites and the number of male sex partners in the past year has implications for the way data on inhalants is collected. The high relationship held for both the men and the women. Whether it is because the men that bisexual women had sex with were also bisexual men who were used to using nitrites, or whether the bisexual women used nitrites to assist in anal intercourse is unclear. In any event, it would seem undesirable to group inhalants such as glue, paint thinner, and gasoline, with the inhalants such as nitrites. The former are not associated with sexual activity, whereas the latter certainly are. These should probably be placed in separate categories for data collection.

We can only state that there is an urgent need for more data to monitor the trends of intravenous drug use in Alaska as this state may soon join others in experiencing an unstoppable epidemic of HIV infection transmitted through this means. We hope that our predictions turn out to be false and that the disaster that we are predicting never takes place. Only time will tell.

REFERENCES

Alaska State Troopers. (1989). *Alaska State Troopers drug report to the Alaska legislature July 1, 1987-June 30, 1988*. Anchorage, AK: State of Alaska, Department of Public Safety (Division of State Troopers).

Booker, J. M., & Hellekson, C. J. (1988, November). *Seasonal affective disorder in Alaska*. Boston, MA: American Public Health Association (Presentation at Annual Conference.

Centers for Disease Control. (1989, March 17). Update: Acquired immunodeficiency syndrome associated with intravenous-drug use-United States, 1988. *Morbidity and Mortality Weekly Report, 38*(10), 165-170.

Centers for Disease Control Task Force on Kaposi's Sarcoma and Opportunistic Infections. (1982). Epidemiologic aspects of the current outbreak of Kaposi's sarcoma and opportunistic infections. *New England Journal of Medicine, 306,* 248-252.

Dicker B.G. (1989). Risk of AIDS among lesbians [Letter to the editor]. *American Journal of Public Health, 79*(11), 1569.

Fisher, D.G., & Brause, J. (1988). *The substance abuse delivery system within the Municipality of Anchorage.* University of Alaska Anchorage. Anchorage, AK: Center for Alcohol and Addiction Studies.

Haverkos, H.W. (1988). Kaposi's Sarcoma and nitrite inhalants. In T.P. Bridge, A.F. Mirsky, & F.K. Goodwin (Eds.), *Psychological, neuropsychiatric, and substance abuse aspects of AIDS* (pp. 165-172). New York: Raven.

Haverkos, H. W., Pinsky, P.F., Drotman, D.P., & Bregman, D.J. (1985). Disease manifestation among homosexual men with acquired immunodeficiency syndrome: A possible role of nitrites in Kaposi's sarcoma. *Sexually Transmitted Diseases, 12,* 203-208.

Howard, C.W., Stovall, K.L., & Farrell, A.D. (1989, August). *Early adolescent sexual behavior: Discriminating factors of sexual health risk-taking.* New Orleans, LA (Paper presented at American Psychological Association).

Identity, Incorporated. (1986). *One in ten: A profile of Alaska's lesbian and gay community.* Anchorage, AK: Author (Box 200070, Anchorage, AK 99520-0070).

Johnson, P.B., & Wilson, P.J. (1988). *Unpublished data.* Anchorage, AK.

Newmeyer, J.A., Feldman, H.W., Biernacki, P., & Watters, J.K. (1989). Preventing AIDS contagion among intravenous drug users. *Medical Anthropology, 10,* 167-175.

Schwarcz, S.K., & Rutherford, G.W. (1989). Acquired immunodeficiency syndrome in infants, children, and adolescents. *The Journal of Drug Issues, 19*(1), 75-92.

Segal, B. (1988). *Drug-taking behavior among Alaskan youth-1988: A follow-up study.* University of Alaska Anchorage. Anchorage, AK: Center for Alcohol and Addiction Studies.

Segal, B., McKelvy, J., Bowman, D., & Mala, T.A. (1983, July 31). *Patterns of drug use: School survey.* Anchorage, AK: Center for Alcohol and Addiction Studies (University of Alaska, Anchorage).

Solomon, M.Z., & DeJong, W. (1989). Preventing AIDS and other STDs through condom promotion: A patient education intervention. *American Journal of Public Health, 79*(4), 453-458.

Stall, R., & Ostrow, D.G. (1989). Intravenous drug use, the combination of drugs and sexual activity and HIV infection among gay and bisexual men: The San Francisco men's health study. *The Journal of Drug Issues, 19*(1), 57-73.

Stall, R., & Wiley, J. (1988). A comparison of alcohol and drug use patterns of homosexual and heterosexual men: The San Francisco Men's Health Study. *Drug and Alcohol Dependence, 22,* 63-73.

Tower, E.A. (1987). Alaska state hepatitis B program: Past, present and future. *Alaska Medicine, 29*(1), 1-8.

Valdiserri, R.O., Arena, V.C., Proctor, D., & Bonati, F.A. (1989). The relationship between women's attitudes about condoms and their use: Implications for condom promotion programs. *American Journal of Public Health, 79*(4), 499-501.

Warning Signs:
Intravenous Drug Abuse
Among American Indians/Alaskan Natives

Ronald M. Rowell, MPH

SUMMARY. The AIDS pandemic has called attention to the existence of intravenous drug abuse among American Indians/Alaskan Natives. Epidemiological data on AIDS and attitudinal surveys provide evidence that IV drug abuse is occurring in American Indian/Alaskan Native communities. There is a need for ongoing research into the prevalence of IV drug abuse in the American Indian/Alaskan Native population. Existing alcoholism treatment programs for Native Americans must be expanded to treat non-alcohol and poly-substance abuse. HIV education and outreach must be initiated with American Indian/Alaskan Native IV drug abusers.

One of the most consistent stereotypes of American Indians and Alaskan Natives is the "drunken Indian," a figure hard to miss in the skid row of almost any major U.S. city. Although not all American Indians/Alaskan Natives are alcoholic, the facts are plain: alcohol accounts for at least four — many would argue the majority — of the top ten causes of death in this population (Congress of the U.S., Office of Technology Assessment, 1986). Intravenous drug abuse on the other hand, is not often thought of in association with American Indians/Alaskan Natives, but there is a growing body of information which is uncovering intravenous drug abuse as a fact of life, at least in some communities.

Ronald M. Rowell (Choctaw/Kaskaskia), is Executive Director of the National Native American AIDS Prevention Center, 6239 College Ave., Suite 201, Oakland, CA 94618.

This center is funded by grant #H62/CCH903122-02 from the U.S. Centers for Disease Control.

The Acquired Immune Deficiency Syndrome pandemic has raised a new — and unmeasured — challenge to professionals in the field of substance abuse serving American Indian/Alaskan Native people. Substance abuse plays a critical role in the transmission of Human Immunodeficiency Virus (HIV), directly through sharing contaminated needles and syringes in intravenous drug abuse, and indirectly through alcohol and non-IV drug abuse and associated risk-taking sexual behavior (Stall, McKusick, Wiley, 1986). The prevalence of alcohol abuse in the Native population is well documented. The prevalence and patterns of intravenous drug abuse are not.

Epidemiological information from the U.S. Centers for Disease Control on cumulative AIDS cases among American Indians/Alaskan Natives provides a glimpse of what may be a larger problem with IV drug abuse in this population than most people realize. As of July 31, 1989, 131 cases of AIDS among American Indians/Alaskan Natives had been reported to the U.S. Centers for Disease Control by at least 22 State Departments of Health in every region of the country. The growth in the number of cases is accelerating. Two American Indian/Alaskan Native AIDS cases had already been diagnosed before 1984 and the cases are roughly doubling every year.

HIV seroprevalence is disproportionately higher for American Indians/Alaskan Natives compared with other groups than is the cumulative incidence of AIDS in the same group (Conway, Hooper, 1989). Data from the HIV antibody testing conducted upon all military recruits by the Department of Defense since October of 1985 indicates a particularly serious problem in California, the state with the largest and most urban American Indian/Alaskan Native population.

Figure 1 shows the prevalence of HIV antibodies in military recruits in the United States as a whole by race/ethnicity (Centers for Disease Control, 1989). It is important to consider that both homosexuals and intravenous drug abusers are assumed to be underrepresented in this sample because of policies denying membership in the Armed Forces to these individuals. American Indian/Alaskan Native military recruits have seropositivity rates above that of White/

FIGURE 1. Seroprevalence of human immunodeficiency virus in U.S. military recruits nationwide by ethnicity, October, 1985 - December, 1988.

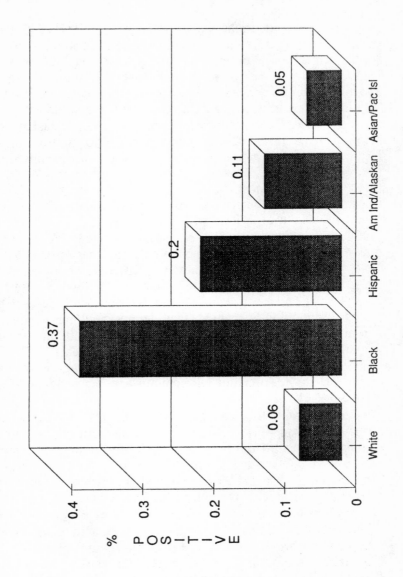

Non-Hispanics and Asian/Pacific Islanders, but below that of Blacks and Hispanics.

In Figure 2, the same study's data for the state of California shows a startling difference between California and the U.S. in the Native American seroprevalence rate. American Indians/Alaskan Natives rank a close second behind Blacks in that state, and far above Hispanics, Whites and Asian/Pacific Islanders. Out of the 908 individuals tested in California, four were seropositive for a rate of 0.44%. Other states with American Indian/Alaskan Native seroprevalence rates equal or higher than California from the military recruit data include Florida (0.81% or one seropositive of 124 tested), Georgia (1.72% or one seropositive of 58 tested), Nevada (1.14% or one seropositive out of 88 tested), New York (0.79% or three seropositives out of 382 tested), and Oregon (0.83% or two seropositives out of 241 tested).

Figure 3 indicates the HIV transmission categories for cumulative American Indian/Alaskan Native AIDS cases through July 31, 1989, in comparison with White/Non-Hispanics. Intravenous drug abuse among American Indian/Alaskan Native AIDS cases, both heterosexual and homosexual, is approximately twice as high as among White/Non-Hispanics. The homosexual/intravenous drug abuser transmission category indicates two exposure modes, either or both of which may have exposed that individual to HIV infection. In any case, it is clear that intravenous drug abuse plays a major role in the spread of HIV among American Indians/Alaskan Natives.

IV drug abuse also accounts for the majority of cases among American Indian/Alaskan Native women and children. Figure 4 indicates the mode of transmission of HIV for mothers of American Indian/Alaskan Native pediatric AIDS cases. As of July 31, 1989, three pediatric cases had been reported. Intravenous drug abuse is responsible for at least two out of the four pediatric cases.

Figure 5 shows clearly that the majority of diagnosed cases of AIDS reported to Centers for Disease Control among American Indian/Alaskan Native women is a result of intravenous drug abuse. Figure 6 breaks down the American Indian/Alaskan Native female cases of AIDS due to heterosexual contact. Although the majority of cases (four out of seven) are undetermined, at least two cases are due to heterosexual contact with an IV drug abuser. It is important

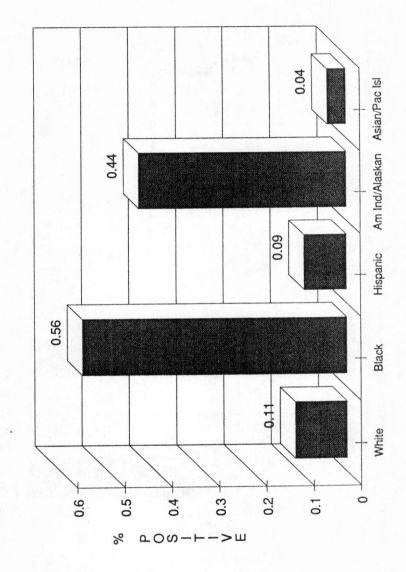

FIGURE 2. Seroprevalence of human immunodeficiency virus in U.S. military recruits in California by ethnicity, October, 1985 - December, 1988.

FIGURE 3. Comparison of human immunodeficiency virus transmission categories between White/Non-Hispanics and American Indians/Alaska Natives. (Homosexual/bisexual, intravenous drug user, homosexual and intravenous drug user, hemophiliac, heterosexual, transfusion recipient, undetermined)

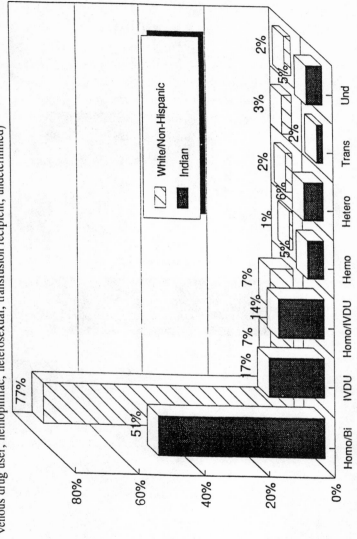

Source: CDC (7/31/89)
N=131

26

FIGURE 4. Human immunodeficiency virus (HIV) transmission categories for mothers of American Indian/Alaskan Native pediatric acquired immune deficiency syndrome cases reported to Centers for Disease Control.

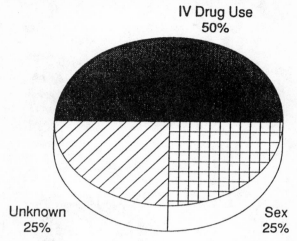

IV Drug Use
50%

Unknown
25%

Sex
25%

Source: CDC (7/31/89)

to note that women make up 18% of the cumulative American Indian/Alaskan Native AIDS caseload, versus only 4% for White/Non-Hispanics.

It is obvious that the key to the prevention of the further spread of HIV among American Indians/Alaskan Natives will be to prevent and to treat substance abuse, both intravenous drug abuse as well as alcohol and other drugs.

Beyond the available epidemiological information on AIDS, there are other studies which point to the spread of IV drug abuse among Native people, and not only in urban areas. A recent study in Alaska for example, indicated that IV drug abuse among Natives is occurring in isolated rural areas (Fisher, Wilson & Brause, in press). That study also reports that Native Alaskans do not appear to be using opiates, choosing instead methamphetamines and cocaine. This information agrees with anecdotal information collected from tribal executives and substance abuse personnel by the National Native American AIDS Prevention Center in northern and southern California and Alaska during 1988. In Vancouver, British Colum-

FIGURE 5. Human immunodeficiency virus transmission categories for Native American women with AIDS reported to the Centers for Disease Control.

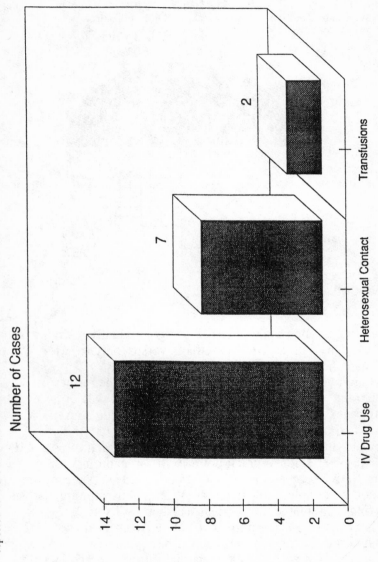

Source: CDC (7/31/89)
N=21

28

FIGURE 6. Sources of human immunodeficiency virus transmission for heterosexual Native American women who were infected through sexual activity.

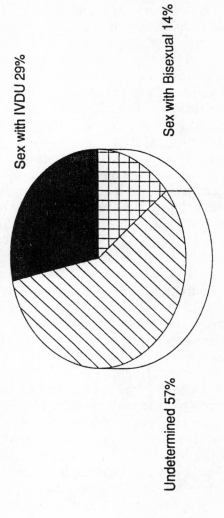

Sex with IVDU 29%

Sex with Bisexual 14%

Undetermined 57%

bia, Canada, a needle-exchange program has reported a range of between 30% and 41% Native Canadian clients per month (Downtown Eastside Youth Activities Society, 1989).

AIDS knowledge, attitudes and behaviors (KAB) surveys in four states of American Indians and Alaska Natives indicate a significant level of IV drug abuse. Although none of these KAB surveys were based upon a probability sample, and inferences regarding the total American Indian/Alaskan Native population must be made with some caution, the information does provide an indication that intravenous drug abuse is a fact of life.

The National Native American AIDS Prevention Center distributed 240 AIDS-related KAB questionnaires to clients in American Indian chemical dependency programs in Minnesota in 1989 (Beaulieu, 1989). One hundred thirty three questionnaires were returned for a response rate of 55.4%. Of the respondents, 56% were male, 41% female. Eighty-five percent of the respondents identified themselves as American Indian. Thirty-eight percent were between the ages of 21 and 30 years, and 26% were between 31 and 40 years old. Forty-six percent of the respondents were reservation residents, 33% were urban, and the rest were rural and small town residents.

The Portland Area Indian Health Board (Hall, White, & Bodenroeder, 1989) surveyed 710 American Indian individuals primarily through tribal agencies and Indian Health Service-funded clinics in the states of Idaho, Washington and Oregon in 1989. Of the 648 who responded to the question, 56% were between the ages of 21 and 40. Seventy-three percent of the 657 respondents to the question on sex were female, and 27% were male. Sixty-six percent of the sample were reservation residents, 34% were non-reservation residents. It is not known how many individuals in the Portland sample may have been in treatment for substance abuse.

Figure 7 illustrates the responses to the question "Have you ever injected (shot) drugs *not* given you by a doctor?" from the Portland study. It is important to remember that the population surveyed in this sample were those attending tribal agencies or IHS-funded primary care clinics. Although comparable data is unavailable for the population at large, the response appears significant to this author, and is greater than most policy makers in the field of American

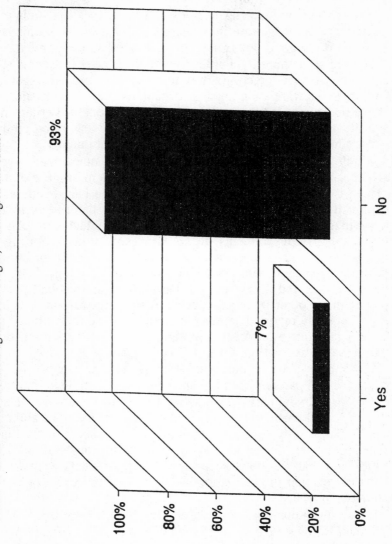

FIGURE 7. Responses to the question: "Have you ever injected (shot) drugs *not* given you by a doctor?" Clients of Indian clinics and tribal agencies in Oregon, Washington and Idaho.

Indian/Alaskan Native substance abuse who focus on the larger problem of alcoholism might assume.

Figure 8 below indicates responses in the Minnesota study to the question "Before getting into treatment, what kinds of things did you *ever* do to get drunk or high? (check all that apply, even if you only tried something)." Thirteen percent of the respondents stated that they had tried injecting drugs at one time or another. Again, the author is unaware of comparable data for non-Native substance abuse programs, but the number appears significant. Perhaps more significant, 30% of the respondents stated that "shooting up drugs (intravenous drug use)" takes place in their community.

Many working in the field of AIDS have questioned whether AIDS should be considered a reservation problem because of a perceived isolation of reservation residents from urban dwellers. The truth is that there is ongoing contact between urban and 11 reservation/village Native people, including sexual contact. For example, of the 71% of respondents in the Minnesota study reporting that they "often" or "sometimes" visited the reservation or city (depending upon their own place of residence), 4% reported that they often had sex and 20% reported that they sometimes had sex with people in the other setting. Sixteen percent of the respondents in the Portland study reported having "moved back and forth often" from the reservation to off-reservation and 51% reported having sexual partners off-reservation. Of the 7% of the study considered at high risk (IV drug abusers and men who have sex with men), 41% reported sexual partners both on- and off-reservation. Over half of the middle-risk individuals (persons with multiple sexual partners) reported sexual partners both on- and off-reservation. The authors of the Portland study concluded that although members of the highest risk group were found a little more often in non-reservation settings, and that middle-risk and low-risk individuals were found a little more often in reservation settings, the differences were very slight.

Sexually transmitted disease rates among American Indians/Alaskan Natives are high compared with U.S. all races and particularly high in some states (Centers for Disease Control, 1985). The interrelationship between Native American STD rates and substance abuse has not been measured, but based upon the work of

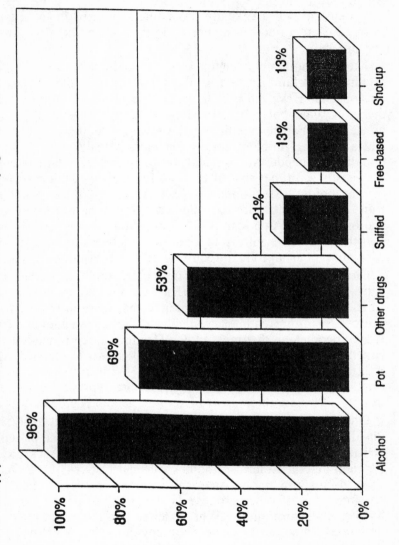

FIGURE 8. Responses to the question: "What kinds of things did you *ever* do to get drunk or high? Answer all that apply." Clients of American Indian substance abuse treatment programs in Minnesota.

33

Stall et al. cited earlier, one should assume a relationship does exist. In the Minnesota KAB study, 25% of the respondents reported that they had had a sexually transmitted disease. In the Portland study, 24% reported having been told they had a sexually transmitted disease.

There is another danger for American Indian/Alaskan Native individuals and families as a result of high rates of diabetes and the existence of HIV: the use of disposable needles and syringes by diabetics which may be reused by IV drug abusers in the same household. Diabetes mellitus is the seventh leading cause of death and a growing problem among the Indian Health Service service population outside Alaska, and the age-adjusted death rate from diabetes is 2.8 times that of U.S. all races (U.S. Congress, Office of Technology Assessment, 1986). Anecdotal information from tribal officials in California collected in informal interviews by the National Native American AIDS Prevention Center in 1988 identified the issue of needle/syringe reuse in diabetic households by IV drug abusers as a problem requiring educational intervention.

Clearly there is an intravenous drug abuse problem among American Indians/Alaskan Natives. What we do not know is how widespread the problem is. We also know that there are very few resources for drug treatment available for American Indian/Alaskan Native people and that most Indian Health Service-funded alcoholism treatment programs are trained only to serve alcoholics, not drug abusers or poly-substance abusers. With the advent of HIV, there is no choice but to act swiftly if we are to prevent unnecessary deaths. There are three areas of activity needing support.

Ongoing research is needed to determine the extent of intravenous drug abuse among Native American people and the patterns of substance abuse in general. Is intravenous drug abuse a growing problem among American Indians/Alaskan Natives? Is the pattern of IV drug abuse among American Indians/Alaskan Natives different from that of other groups? Is the problem limited to certain locales, states or regions? What external variables may play a part in the pattern of substance abuse in any given locale? What are the intravenous drugs of choice and do they differ from place to place? We must be able to answer these and other related questions if we are to develop strategies to save Native lives.

Existing Native alcoholism treatment programs must be expanded to enable the treatment of other types of substance abuse. They must integrate HIV prevention education into the overall treatment plan. The number of treatment programs and slots available must be expanded if we are serious about improving the health status of American Indian/Alaskan Native people and preventing unnecessary deaths.

Local communities should be encouraged to involve ex-IV drug abusers in an effort to prevent the spread of AIDS through information, education and bleach distribution for cleaning needles for intravenous drug abusers not in treatment. Needle exchange programs should be carefully evaluated and considered by local communities. Nothing less than an immediate, coordinated effort to expose and treat the problem of IV drug abuse among Native Americans will help stop HIV.

REFERENCES

Beaulieu, L. (1989). *American Indian chemical dependency treatment program AIDS-related knowledge, attitudes and behavior survey*. Oakland, CA: National Native American AIDS Prevention Center.

Centers for Disease Control, AIDS Program. (1989). *Prevalence of HIV-1 antibody in civilian applicants for military service by state, sex and ethnic group, October, 1985-December, 1988*. Unpublished raw data.

Congress of the United States, Office of Technology Assessment. (1986). *Indian health care* (Publication No. OTA-H-290). Washington, DC: U.S. Government Printing Office.

Conway, G., & Hooper, E.Y. (1989, June). *Risk of AIDS and HIV infection in American Indians and Alaska Natives*. Poster session presented at the 5th International Conference on AIDS, Montreal.

Downtown Eastside Youth Activities Society. (1989). *First Report of the City-Funded Needle Exchange Program*. Vancouver, BC: John Bardsley.

Fisher, D.G., Wilson, P.J., & Brause, J. (in press). Intravenous drug use in Alaska. *Psychology of Addictive Behaviors*.

Hall, R., White, D., & Bodenroeder, P. (1989). *A Survey of knowledge, attitudes, and behaviors related to AIDS among Native Americans of Oregon, Idaho and Washington*. Portland, OR: Northwest Portland Area Indian Health Board.

Stall, R., McKusick, L., & Wiley, J. (1986). Alcohol and drug use during sexual activity and compliance with safe sex guidelines for AIDS: The AIDS Behavioral Research Project. *Health Education Quarterly*, *13*, 359-371.

The Human Immunodeficiency Virus in Alaska and Its Relationship to Intravenous Drug Use

Dennis Leoutsakas, MA

SUMMARY. There is a distinct relationship between the Human Immunodeficiency Virus (HIV) and Intravenous Drug (IVD) use. The low number of cases of the HIV reported in Alaska makes it important to realize the extent of the IVD using population in the state to determine the depth of the health problem. Once identified, IVD users with the HIV present some educational, treatment, and ethical dilemmas for care providers. Current and accurate information is essential to Alaskan communities, and Alaskan agencies must take a more active role in changing attitudes, while seeking updated information.

The impact of the HIV is becoming clearer as we continue to use demographic and geographic means to monitor the spread of the infection. In the United States, the rural states, as can be expected, are experiencing fewer cases than those with major urban centers. Alaska, with a population under 500,00 is therefore rated among the ten states reporting the lowest number of cases of the Acquired Immune Deficiency Syndrome (AIDS) (Centers for Disease Control [CDC], 1989, April). The Alaska Department of Epidemiology has reported that 256 people have tested positive for the HIV through the State Public Health Laboratories, and there are 65 confirmed cases of AIDS in the state (Section of Epidemiology, 1989, February 3). Fewer than 10 of the state's reported AIDS cases are identified as IVD users, and only 16 of the 12,936 persons tested through

Dennis Leoutsakas is affiliated with the National Association of People with AIDS (Alaska), P.O. Box 240405, Anchorage, AK 99524.

the state Public Health Laboratories were both IVD users and infected with the HIV. Keeping the low incidence in mind, this paper will discuss locating the IVD users in Alaska and take a more detailed look at the prevention, education, and treatment strategies used by community-based organizations and the State of Alaska to address the HIV in relationship to the IVD users. Within this framework, the paper will also focus on some ethical questions that both Alaska and the nation must face as the health care community continues to confront this relatively new and enigmatic virus.

DEFINITIONS

The terms defined in this section are included to provide consistency throughout the article.

Human immunodeficiency virus (HIV). The HIV is a specific virus that attacks the immune system and decreases it's ability to defend against opportunistic conditions. AIDS is included within the parameters of this definition and will be reflected in the discussion as a separate entity only when indicated otherwise by research.

Intravenous drug (IVD). An IVD is any illicit drug that is injected directly into the blood stream. No distinction is made between drugs that can be taken either intravenously or intramuscularly.

Intravenous drug user (IVD user). Any person who has injected, or is injecting, illicit drugs on a regular basis and/or in an unsterile manner is an IVD user. Two or more times in a year is regular usage. Any differences between active IVD users and recovering IVD users is noted in the discussion.

At risk. Any time people share IVDs in an unsterile environment is considered "at risk."

FINDING THE IVD USER

Rarely in modern times is it in the best interest of IVD users to advertise their use of illicit drugs, and all 50 states have laws making the use of a variety of drugs illegal. To avoid the possibility of arrest, and incarceration, most IVD users will not openly acknowledge their drug use. The legal realities plus the social stigma attached to IVD use create a subculture of active IVD users and addicts who remain distanced from "mainstream" society. Similarly, recovering IVD users are often unwilling to openly discuss their drug histories to protect themselves from the possibility of discrimination. It is difficult therefore, to locate the IVD users, both present and past, within the general population.

Until recently, IVD use in Alaska has been minimally discussed in studies, and ignored in the open literature (Fisher, Wilson, & Brause, in press). Current annual reports from the Alaska State Office of Alcoholism and Drug Abuse have categorized statistics by type of drug rather than by the route of administration (State Office of Alcoholism and Drug Abuse [SOADA], 1988, 1989). Other studies focus on small segments of the population, but fail to isolate the total subculture of IVD users specifically (Segal, 1988; Segal, McKelvy, Bowman, & Mala, 1983, July 31). One reason for the neglect of the IVD users in research, may be the difficulty in finding the IVD users among the general population.

The HIV has been entrenched in the United States since 1981, and we know that there were cases of AIDS reported as early as 1969 and 1977 (Shilts, 1987; Shoumatoff, 1988, July). Any active or recovering IVD user that has used IVD's since the early 1970s is potentially infected by the HIV. There are a large number of drugs that can be taken intravenously. The most common IVD's are heroin, cocaine, and amphetamines, but there is an imposing group of others such as a number of other opium derivatives, and a variety of pharmaceuticals that are suitable for injection. In Alaska there is a particular problem with Dilaudid (Fisher et al., in press). An active or recovering IVD user may have used any number of drugs and is at risk of infection.

In relation to the HIV, it is time for health care organizations in the State of Alaska to locate the IVD using population, both past and present, and target them for special education and prevention activities. The emphasis of the education and prevention should be on infection control, but may include substance abuse information and treatment referrals when suitable. A role for researchers in Alaska is to determine the extent of the IVD use in the state and to direct both State agencies and community based organizations to areas, groups, and people with the highest risk of infection from the HIV.

EDUCATION

Providing adequate education about the HIV to IVD users in Alaska is proving to be a difficult task. The size of the state and its rural nature are increasing the difficulty in locating persons at risk of infection from the HIV. Only Anchorage, with a population of 220,000 and Fairbanks with a population of 70,000, have developed programs to specifically address the HIV among active IVD users within their cities (Narcotic Drug Treatment Center [NDTC], 1988, June 30). There are indications also that only a minimal amount of information is reaching rural areas outside of the three main urban centers of Anchorage, Fairbanks, and Juneau (J. Palmer, personal communication, May 30, 1989). Provisions for continuing education for health care workers outside these three cities is sparse and some rural health care providers are unwilling to provide HIV antibody testing (J. E. Nichols, personal communication, January, 1989).

To provide a minimum amount of education and prevention information to Alaskan communities is counting on a low probability of infection. It does not take into consideration small pockets of people at risk, nor does it consider the real possibility of an unexpected outbreak of the virus. It also does not prepare families and health care providers to care for someone in the later stages of infection who may enter or re-enter their communities. There has been a significant increase in the number of IVD users testing positive for the HIV through the state public health laboratories (Section of Epidemiology, 1989, February 3). In December 1987 there were 9 reported cases of positive test results among 766 identified IVD users in the state, and by December of 1988 that number had risen to 16 out of 1,060 tested (Section of Epidemiology, 1987, December, 1989, February 3).

The State Office of Alcohol and Drug Abuse (SOADA), Alaska's primary funding source for public drug and alcohol prevention and treatment programs is developing a training plan that provides for a comprehensive curriculum and ongoing education in an effort to respond to these recent data (Armstrong, 1989). To date, the state has not implemented a formal policy to specifically address the HIV among IVD users. It seems essential that the state legislature fund a program as soon as possible in an effort to curtail the continued spread of the HIV among the IVD using population, and to lessen the chances of the virus being transmitted to the general population by IVD users.

TREATING THE DUALLY DIAGNOSED

A person is diagnosed with the HIV when they either test positive for antibodies to the virus, or when they display symptoms that show the virus is compromising the immune system. Public health agencies generally use the ELISA and the Western Blot to screen blood for antibodies to the HIV, and combined positive test results are considered to be greater than 99% accurate (Centers for Disease Control [CDC], 1988, January 8). A diagnosis of IVD use is a little more difficult to assess. A diagnostician must consider: (a) the length of time since last injection, (b) the total number of injections, and (c) the frequency of injections before categorizing a person as an IVD user.

A diagnosis of IVD use is further complicated by trying to define the difference between active use, and past use. There are many persons in various stages of recovery and a large segment of the recovering population still consider themselves to be addicts (Narcotics Anonymous [NA], 1989). Most diagnoses for IVD use are made upon intake at a health care facility or a treatment center.

Treatment for people with a dual diagnosis of HIV infection and IVD use is problematic in Alaska. Persons with the HIV encounter substance abuse treatment systems that are unprepared, or unwilling to work with them (Armstrong, 1989). Persons with AIDS, who are experiencing medical complications, have even fewer options for substance abuse treatment available to them. Treatment centers which have accepted HIV seropositive clients in the past found that those infected have a difficult time focusing on their substance use, and staff are unable to guide their client(s) to successful completion of the programs (J. Morgan, personal communication, January, 1989). HIV infected, recovering IVD users who attend outpatient groups and 12-step programs often feel stigmatized, and fail to attend or participate if they are identified (Ainlay, Becker, & Coleman, 1986).

Active IVD users who seek to address only the HIV and ignore their substance use often use the virus to deny their involvement with illicit drugs. The denial can cause an array of problems for the person's health care providers, and public health officials. A person with the HIV who continues to use IVDs can experience medical difficulties, social conflicts (especially with family members), psychological and emotional problems, and moral dilemmas. The problems can eventually lead to death.

In Alaska there has been limited training available for those treating the dually diagnosed. A low known incidence rate of people infected with the HIV, and a low number of cases of AIDS reported, has created little demand for education among substance abuse counselors. Adequately trained and knowledgeable persons, who can act as resources need to be strategically located throughout the state, and health care professionals and substance abuse counselors need access to updated and accurate information so that they may take a more active role when working with someone who has a dual diagnosis. Because there are so few known cases, opportunities arise for care providers to prepare extensive treatment plans for continued care of their clients without being overwhelmed by an unmanageable number of cases. To prepare Alaska to meet the challenges presented by the dually diagnosed, program administrators must review current policies for communicable diseases and issues such as housing, employment, hospitalization, insurance, and ongoing education will have to be addressed or incorporated.

ETHICAL DILEMMAS

Are aggressive prevention and education strategies the keys to controlling the spread of the HIV among the IVD using population? If so, how much time and money should be spent for treatment of a person diagnosed with AIDS? Are needle exchange programs subtly advocating for continued drug use? If a person is identified as infected with the HIV upon an initial assessment and the person is an active IVD user, what are the obligations of the screener? Should treatment centers deny persons who have the HIV access to their programs? All these questions, and more, open a "Pandora's box" of ethical dilemmas for substance abuse counselors and health care workers. The issues are not unique to Alaska, but are also being felt on a national level (Des Jarlais, Jainchill, & Friedman, 1988; Ginzburg & Gostin, 1988).

An attempt to discuss all the ethical dilemmas faced by Alaskan health care workers is unrealistic. There are, however, some issues that are being confronted by professionals as they continue to work with IVD users at risk for infection with the HIV. Anchorage, for instance, has a program intended to provide outreach services to active IVD users. The majority of their outreach workers are former IVD users. It makes sense to use a member of an identified subculture to work with the specific members of the group, but the outreach workers are subjecting themselves to continued pressure to begin using illicit drugs again. The result of the pressure is that many of the program's outreach workers are returning to substance use (P. Johnson, personal communication, March, 1989). The price of educating the IVD using population about the HIV using this method seems too high, and the program will need to develop other prevention and intervention strategies similar to those used by older and more established programs (Friedman, Des Jarlais, & Sotheran, 1988).

Historically, substance abuse programs have asserted the privilege of refusing treatment to potential clients. Often this is the case when a program considers people unsuitable for treatment or a threat to the milieu. Waiting lists for reasonably-priced treatment programs are also a temporary deterrent for admission to a facility. Refusing treatment to people who are infected with the HIV limits their options for rehabilitation, and sets the stage for continued drug use. For IVD users who are infected, this often means putting others at risk for infection from the HIV. The price for productive, or successful treatment programs therefore, is the risk of continued infection among the IVD using population. The American Medical Society on Alcoholism and Other Drug Dependencies [AMSAODD] (1988, June), private agencies, and others (Beauchamp, 1986, April) throughout the United States have all begun to address this ethical dilemma faced by programs for the chemically dependent (Gostin, 1988). Alaskan agencies need to follow suit and upgrade their current policies and procedures so that they meet the challenges presented by HIV-infected and chemically-dependent persons, and respond to the potential health crises within the communities they serve.

Free needle programs and needle exchange programs are a continuous source of controversy. Many people think that the programs will help to control the spread of the HIV, while others believe that the needle programs subtly support illicit drug use. Alaska has yet to have to face this ethical dilemma publicly, and most of the discussions about needle programs have been philosophical to date. It would be insightful of the State Office of Alcoholism and Drug Abuse to establish a policy addressing such programs because there is a growing support for them within the health community (Anonymous, 1989, April 10; Ginzburg & Gostin, 1988).

Disbursement of available money is another complex issue. In the rapidly expanding AIDS industry it seems as if more and more people and agencies are seeking funds. This leads to insufficient funding for all service providers and a dilemma for grantors. This issue is not unique to Alaska and health care providers throughout the nation are beginning to address the inequities fostered by our health care system (Cooperman, 1989, June 4). Alaska is already experiencing financial strain on its public health care system, and the inclusion of people infected with the HIV can only be expected to add greater stress. Under the present health care system, grantors need to appropriate money carefully with special consideration for the areas of research, treatment, and education/prevention. Disbursed funds should also meet the specific needs of the Alaskan communities they are directed to, and the present health care system should be upgraded if it is failing to provide adequate services.

CONCLUSION

Alaska, in comparison with many states, is aggressively attacking the issues that surround both the HIV and the IVD use in the state. Until recently, however, the state has treated the issues as separate ones and efforts were seldom coordinated. In an attempt to control the spread of the HIV among the IVD population in Alaska, researchers and agencies collecting data need to locate and identify IVD users to determine the extent of the HIV infected population. Research should be done in a collaborative effort with treatment providers and educators, so that providers can offer practical treatment to those in need and educators can design effective forums for teaching. Both the HIV and IVD use are family diseases, and education should be directed to whole families when possible. Training plans for rural areas of Alaska need to prepare health care professionals and health aides for the impact of the HIV on their small communities. Also families and friends of those infected need to learn how to create and utilize support systems for themselves as they prepare to care for their loved ones.

To effectively treat the dually diagnosed persons in Alaska is to understand the breadth of the diagnosis. It includes people who have not been at risk for years, and it also includes active IVD users. The diagnosis also includes an array of drugs that are commonly labeled *other* in research projects. Treatment specialists, and health care professionals need to be cross-trained to handle the many issues that can arise from the diverse population they will encounter. Treatment centers, residential settings, outpatient clinics, and 12-step programs can expect to confront issues and problems that were previously ignored or unknown.

For the IVD user infected with the HIV, current and accurate information is an essential ingredient for adequate and successful treatment. It also provides a firm foundation for resolving the ethical dilemmas that are surfacing. Care providers in Alaska must ensure that there is a continuous flow of information into the state if they hope to meet the challenges before them.

REFERENCES

Ainlay, S. C., Becker, G., & Coleman, L. M. (Eds.). (1986). *The dilemma of difference*. New York: Plenum.
American Medical Society on Alcoholism and Other Drug Dependencies. (1988, June). *Guidelines for facilities treating chemically dependent patients at risk for AIDS or infected by HIV virus*. New York: Author.
Anonymous. (1989, April 10). Needle exchange?: A drastic plan whose time may have come, if limited, legal and tied to drug rehabilitation [Editorial]. *San Francisco Chronicle*.

Armstrong, M. (1989). *SOADA plan for AIDS related substance abuse training*. Anchorage, AK: State Office of Alcohol and Drug Abuse.

Beauchamp, D. (1986, April). AIDS and alcoholism: The parallels. *Acquired immune deficiency syndrome and chemical dependency*, pp. 43-52 (DHHS Publication No. (ADM) 88-1513).

Centers for Disease Control. (1988, January 8). Update: Serologic testing for antibody to Human Immunodeficiency Virus. *Morbidity and Mortality Weekly Report*, 36(52), 833-839.

Centers for Disease Control. (1989, April). AIDS cases reported through March 1989. *HIV/AIDS Surveillance Report*, pp. 1-16.

Cooperman, A. (1989, June 4). U.S. health care system unfair, Koop asserts. *Anchorage Daily News*, p. A4.

Des Jarlais, D. C., Jainchill, N., & Friedman, S. R. (1988). AIDS among IV drug users: Epidemiology, natural history, and therapeutic community experiences. In R. P. Galea, B. F. Lewis, & L. A. Baker (Eds.), *AIDS and IV drug abusers: Current perspectives* (pp. 51-60). Owings Mills, MD: National Health.

Fisher, D. G., Wilson, P. J., & Brause, J. (in press). Intravenous drug use in Alaska. *Drugs and Society*.

Friedman, S. R., Des Jarlais, D. C., & Sotheran, J. L. (1988). AIDS health education for intravenous drug users. In R. P. Galea, B. F. Lewis, & L. A. Baker (Eds.), *AIDS and IV drug abusers: Current perspectives* (pp. 199-214). Owings Mills, MD: National Health.

Ginzburg, H. M., & Gostin, L. (1988). Legal and ethical issues associated with HIV disease. In R. P. Galea, B. F. Lewis, & L. A. Baker (Eds.), *AIDS and IV drug abusers: Current perspectives* (pp. 243-252). Owings Mills, MD: National Health.

Gostin, L. (1988). Drug-dependent populations: Legal and public policy options. In R. P. Galea, B. F. Lewis, & L. A. Baker (Eds.), *AIDS and IV drug abusers: Current perspectives* (pp. 253-265). Owings Mills: MD: National Health.

Narcotic Drug Treatment Center. (1988, June 30). *Annual report*. Anchorage, AK: Center for Drug Problems.

Narcotics Anonymous. (1989). *Narcotics anonymous*. Leetonia, OH: World Service Conference (Literature Sub-Committee).

Section of Epidemiology. (1987, December). *Quarterly report for the State of Alaska AIDS Program*. Anchorage, AK: State of Alaska (Department of Health and Social Services).

Section of Epidemiology. (1989, February 3). Through December 31, 1988. *State of Alaska Epidemiology Bulletin*, p. 1 (Department of Health and Social Services).

Segal, B. (1988). *Drug-taking behavior among Alaskan youth-1988: A follow-up study*. Anchorage, AK: Center for Alcohol and Addiction Studies.

Segal, B., McKelvy, J., Bowman, D., & Mala, T. A. (1983, July 31). *Patterns of drug use: School survey*. Anchorage, AK: Center for Alcohol and Addiction Studies. (University of Alaska, Anchorage).

Shilts, R. (1987). *And the band played on*. New York: St. Martin's.

Shoumatoff, A. (1988, July). In search of the source. *Vanity Fair*, pp. 95-117.

State Office of Alcoholism and Drug Abuse. (1988). *Annual report to the legislature*. Juneau, AK: State of Alaska (AK/DHSS/SOADA/89-3).

State Office of Alcoholism and Drug Abuse. (1989). *The economic cost of alcohol and other drug abuse in Alaska*. Juneau, AK: State of Alaska (AK/DHSS/SOADA/89-1).

Drinking, Alcoholism, and Sexual Behavior in a Cohort of Gay Men

John L. Martin, PhD, MPH
Deborah S. Hasin, PhD

SUMMARY. The relationships between usual alcohol consumption, alcoholism, and sexual behavior were examined using data derived from a sample of 604 New York City gay men who had been interviewed annually in 1985, 1986, and 1987, and who did not have a diagnosis of AIDS. Alcohol consumption was measured as the product of usual quantity and frequency of drinking over the year prior to each interview. Diagnoses of alcohol abuse and dependence during the years of 1986 and 1987 were assessed using the National Institute of Mental Health (NIMH) Diagnostic Interview Schedule (DIS). Sexual behaviors varied in their risk of transmission of Human Immunodeficiency Virus (HIV), (the cause of Acquired Immunodeficiency Syndrome [AIDS]), and included insertive and receptive oral-genital sex and unprotected insertive and receptive anal intercourse. Significant associations were found between usual alcohol consumption and oral sex in 1985 and 1986, but not in 1987. Those identified as alcoholic also reported significantly more epi-

---

John L. Martin is Assistant Professor and Deborah S. Hasin is Research Scientist at the Columbia University College of Physicians and Surgeons, Department of Psychiatry and School of Public Health, Division of Sociomedical Sciences, 600 West 168 Street, New York, NY 10032.

This research was supported by grant MH39557 from the National Institute of Mental Health and by the New York City Department of Health. The authors also acknowledge the support of the New York State Department of Mental Hygiene, and NIMH grant MH30906-07 for computer support. Thanks to Laura Dean for her helpful comments on earlier drafts of the manuscript. Also, thanks to Sean Symons for his statistical work and computer services.

Address reprint requests to John L. Martin, Columbia University School of Public Health, 600 West 168 Street, New York, NY 10032.

© 1991 by The Haworth Press, Inc. All rights reserved.

sodes of receptive oral sex in 1987. No other significant associations were found. This pattern of results did not change when lover status and age were controlled for as covariates. These results are discussed in light of their implications for future work on the issue of drinking and sexual risk taking.

As the AIDS epidemic continues to expand beyond 100,000 cases in the U.S., the determinants of sexual behavior and drug injecting behavior have become topics of intensive study (Turner, Miller & Moses, 1989). Reducing the rates of these behaviors, which are responsible for over 90% of all AIDS cases, has become a major undertaking by health agencies at all levels of government, from the U.S. Public Health Service Centers for Disease Control (CDC) to state and city public health clinics and grass roots community groups. To the extent that key factors can be identified which are responsible for promoting or deterring behavior that transmits Human Immunodeficiency Virus (HIV) these public health efforts can be expanded and enhanced.

Alcohol has been shown to play an important role in both sexual arousal and sexual aggression. (See Crowe & George, 1989 for a recent review of this literature.) In addition, drinking is believed to lead to the disinhibition of behaviors normally kept in check by personal and social standards of conduct (Room & Collins, 1983). It is thus not surprising that a number of researchers working in the area of behavioral aspects of HIV disease and AIDS have focused on drinking and alcohol use as a potential target for study. The most developed work in this field has been reported by Stall and colleagues (Stall, 1988; Stall, McKusick, Wiley, Coates & Ostrow, 1986). These researchers, studying both drug and alcohol use, demonstrated that drinking while engaging in sexual behavior was significantly associated with higher risk sexual activities in a sample of San Francisco gay men. In a more recent report (Stall, 1989) additional data were presented from two other samples of gay men in San Francisco which appeared to corroborate the earlier findings and support the hypothesis that drinking is associated with risk taking during sexual behavior.

Findings from other investigations, however, are less consistent and suggest a more complex association between alcohol consumption and sexual behavior. For example, Cooper, Skinner, George and Brunner (1989) studied the role of drinking among heterosexual adolescents in order to evaluate the role of alcohol in promoting unplanned pregnancies and HIV transmission. Significant associations between alcohol and casual partners, condom use, and communication between partners, were found only with regard to the *first* occasion of intercourse. The relationship between drinking alcohol and these risk-related aspects of sex appeared to diminish with subsequent episodes of intercourse.

Doll (1989) studied the determinants of unprotected oral and anal sex among urban gay men from Chicago, Denver, and San Francisco. She found that although the use of multiple drugs (including alcohol) was significantly associated with higher risk sexual activities alcohol consumption, alone, was not. Nor was a treatment history for alcoholism found to be associated with high risk sexual activity.

The idea that the association between drinking and risk taking during sex may be complex is further supported by the fact that alcohol consumption influences sexual behavior through both psychological and physical pathways, and these effects may be antagonistic with respect to sexual arousal and performance (see Crowe & George, 1989, for a recent review). That is, the physical effect of increasing doses of alcohol is to suppress sexual responding while the effects of increasing doses on psychological processes may promote sexual responsiveness and subsequent behavior through the impairment of learned inhibitions, damaged cognitive capabilities, and a variety of attributional biases.

A complete understanding of the relation between drinking and risk taking may also require the integration of theory and findings from the literature on the role of alcohol expectancies in determining behavior (Briddell & Wilson, 1976; Critchlow, 1983, 1986; MacAndrew & Edgerton, 1969). Despite a variety of methodological and conceptual problems with this research (see Leigh, 1989), the available evidence supports the idea that established beliefs about alcohol's effects are significant determinants of behavior occurring under the influence of alcohol. Although many individuals hold the expectation that alcohol will intensify their sexual experiences, make them more sexually responsive, romantic, and less shy

(Athanasiou, Shaver & Tavris, 1970; Rockwell, Ellinwood & Kantor, 1973), it is not at all clear that similar expectations exist with regard to risk taking during sex. This may be particularly important to consider when studying the link between drinking and sexual risk taking in populations where attractive options for safer sexual behavior exist and have had the time to become socially accepted and approved, as they have been among many gay men. For such populations drinking may indeed be associated with increased sexual activity considered to be safe, but may not be associated with sexual activities considered to be risky, or unsafe. Thus, when investigating possible links between risk taking during sex and alcohol consumption, it may be useful to have distinct measures of behaviors ranging from high risk activities to low risk activities.

The purpose of the present study was to examine the association between alcohol consumption and sexual behavior in a cohort of gay men drawn from the gay community of New York City. Our primary aim was to test the hypothesis that higher levels of alcohol consumption would be related to increased rates of sexual behavior. In order to evaluate the specificity of this hypothesis with regard to risk taking, we focused on sexual behaviors that varied along two dimensions.

The first dimension involved high risk versus low risk sexual behaviors. Epidemiologic studies have clearly established unprotected receptive anal intercourse as the sexual activity which carries the highest risk for HIV infection (Chmiel et al., 1987; Kingsley et al., 1987; Martin, Garcia, & Beatrice, 1989; Mayer et al., 1986; Moss et al., 1987; Stevens et al., 1986; Winkelstein, Lyman & Padian, 1987) and AIDS (Jaffe et al., 1983; Polk et al., 1987) in the gay male population. In contrast, receptive or insertive oral-genital sex, with or without a condom, has not been shown to carry a high degree of risk of HIV infection, and thus is considered by many gay men to be low risk.

The second dimension represented in the present measures involved the distinction between imposing risk on another versus taking risk upon one's self. This distinction is clearly an important one from the standpoint of HIV transmission. As noted above the risk of infection clearly increases with the frequency of being the receptive partner during intercourse, but it does not increase with the frequency of insertive episodes. While little work has been done on the determinants of being the insertive versus the receptive partner during sex among gay men, it seemed important to separate these two aspects of risk when studying the role of alcohol in sexual behavior, because drinking may influence one aspect of risk but not the other; that is, drinking may be associated with higher rates of imposing risk on others but may not affect the rate of taking risk upon one's self, or vice versa.

In addition to representing different aspects of risk taking, it also seemed important to measure alcohol consumption in multiple ways, as there is little consistency in the measurement of drinking across studies. One simple approach involves assessment of usual drinking patterns or number of drinks imbibed in a given amount of time. The behavioral clarity of such a measure makes it attractive, both conceptually and methodologically. However, similar amounts of alcohol do not affect all individuals in the same way: A phenomenon which is ignored by a strictly behavioral approach to the measurement of drinking. Thus, it also seemed useful to identify a group of individuals who clearly had problems due to excessive drinking, without attempting to impose a specific cut off point for defining *excessive drinking*. To accomplish this, we took a diagnostic approach in which individuals were assessed for the presence of symptoms of alcohol dependence and alcohol abuse.

METHOD

Study Participants and Data Collection

In 1985 746 gay male residents of New York City, aged 20 to 70 who did not have AIDS, were recruited through one of two steps in the sampling process. First, an initial pool of 291 men (39%) were recruited directly by the researchers through the following channels: (1) Gay organizations ($n = 131$), (2) unsolicited volunteers ($n = 41$), (3) pilot sample referrals ($n = 32$), (4) the 1985 New York City Gay Pride Festival ($n = 72$), and (5) a public health clinic ($n = 15$). The remaining 455 (61%) respondents were recruited through personal referrals to the study by those 291 already interviewed.

Following the baseline interview at wave 1 in 1985, two follow-up interviews were conducted with respondents at one year intervals, in 1986 and 1987. Respondents who failed to complete all three interviews or who developed AIDS during the course of the study were not included in this analysis. As of 1987, 604 respondents (81% of the original sample) had been interviewed three times and had not been diagnosed with AIDS. The panel sample (N = 604) was relatively unchanged compared with the original sample. Respondents were primarily White (89%), college educated (72%), Manhattan residents (74%), with a median income of $30,000 in 1986, and a mean age of 38 in 1987. Forty two percent of the respondents were coupled with a lover. (A respondent qualified as having a lover if (a) he said he had a lover; (b) his lover viewed him as his lover [reciprocity]; (c) friends viewed the two as a couple [public recognition]; and (d) the relationship was extant for six months or more [duration].)

Structured interviews were conducted in respondents' homes. Interviews lasted from two to four hours with sections administered to subjects in a standardized order. Identical questions were asked about drug use and sexual behavior in each annual interview. The time frame covered by each interview was the 12 months prior to the interview. Because interviews were conducted in the middle of each year, the 1985 data reflect activity from mid-1984 to mid-1985, the 1986 data reflect activity from mid-1985 to mid-1986, and the 1987 data reflect activity from mid-1986 to mid-1987.

The interviewer team consisted of 10 to 13 men and women and included both gay and non-gay individuals. No interviewer effects have been detected to date on any of the variables used in this analysis. Written informed consent was obtained from all participants in accordance with procedures approved by the Columbia Presbyterian Medical Center Institutional Review Board.

MEASURES

Usual Alcohol Consumption

Usual consumption of alcohol was measured as the product of (a) the frequency of drinking in a typical week during the year prior to the interview (response options ranged from 0 [never] to 4 [daily]) and (b) the usual number of drinks consumed per episode of drinking (maximum response option = 5). The resulting product ranged from zero (no alcohol for the year) to 20 (daily consumption of five or more drinks for the year). The average score on this measure was highly stable across all three waves of data: 1984-85 M = 3.6, SD = 3.3; 1985-86 M = 3.6, SD = 3.8; 1986-87 M = 3.7, SD = 3.5. In addition, the proportion of the panel sample abstaining from drinking was also stable across the three waves of data: 15.3%, 16.1%, and 15.9%. (See Martin, 1990a, for a discussion of these trends.)

Current Alcoholism

In order to determine current status regarding alcohol abuse or alcohol dependence we included the alcohol section of the NIMH Diagnostic Interview Schedule (DIS) version 3 (Robins, Helzer, Ratcliff & Seyfried, 1982) as part of the larger interview for wave 2 (1985-86) and wave 3 (1986-87). This instrument was designed for use by non-clinician interviewers. The DIS assesses diagnoses of lifetime alcohol abuse and alcohol dependence according to criteria from the Diagnostic and Statistical Manual, third edition (DSM-III; American Psychiatric Association, 1980). According to the standard DIS procedures, the most recent occurrence of any alcohol problem reported in the interview determines the recency of the disorder. We defined *current* as recency within the last year. Several studies have shown that among all psychiatric diagnoses, DIS diagnoses of alcohol or drug abuse/dependence agree best with assessments made by mental health professionals (Hasin & Grant, 1987; Helzer et al., 1985; Robins et al., 1984). In the present sample the prevalence of current DIS/DSM-III alcoholism for wave 2 (1985-86) was 12.1% (73/604); for wave 3 (1986-87) the prevalence was 9.3% (56/604) (Martin, 1990a; Martin, Dean, Garcia & Hall, 1989).

Sexual Behavior

Oral Sex

The annual frequency of engaging in oral-genital sex was determined separately for receptive and insertive activity. The measures were derived by weighting the total number of sexual episodes for the year by the proportion of those episodes during which each type of oral sex was performed (Martin, 1987). Although we inquired about oral-genital sex both with and without a condom, the use of condoms during oral sex was too rare to generate stable estimates (Martin, Dean, Garcia & Hall, 1989). Thus, we did not conduct analyses involving condom protected oral sex.

Unprotected Anal Intercourse

The annual frequency of engaging in unprotected anal intercourse was determined separately for receptive intercourse and insertive intercourse. The measures (see Martin [1987] for a complete description) were derived as follows: First, the number of sexual episodes in which the respondent engaged in each type of anal intercourse was determined. Second, the proportion of these episodes during which a condom was used was determined and transformed into a frequency value for condom-protected intercourse episodes. Third, the number of protected intercourse episodes was subtracted from the total number of episodes. Thus, respondents who either never engaged in [receptive/insertive] anal intercourse during a given year, or who "always" used a condom when they engaged in anal intercourse during that year received a score of zero (0). Respondents who "never" used a condom when they engaged in [receptive/insertive] anal intercourse received a score equal to the number of times they engaged in the particular type of anal intercourse during that year.

The average annual frequency for the panel sample of engaging in each type of sexual behavior is shown in Table 1. Prior analyses have shown that the decreases over time in the frequency of each type of sexual act are statistically significant (Martin, Dean, Garcia & Hall, 1989). In addition, the distributions of these variables are highly positively skewed (Martin, 1987; Martin, Dean, Garcia & Hall, 1989). Thus, a log transformation was applied to each variable prior to conducting statistical tests in order to better meet the assumptions of the prediction models. However, for descriptive analyses we present raw means and standard deviations.

Table 1

Average Annual Frequency (SD) of Engaging in Four Types of Sexual

Behaviors

Sexual behavior	Year		
	1984-85	1985-86	1986-87
Receptive oral-genital sex	50.5 (69.8)	41.1 (60.2)	36.7 (60.5)
Insertive oral-genital sex	49.3 (61.6)	42.0 (60.4)	34.6 (56.1)
Unprotected receptive anal intercourse	16.5 (39.3)	7.1 (23.1)	5.6 (27.9)
Unprotected insertive anal intercourse	20.9 (47.4)	10.3 (29.8)	6.1 (22.5)

57

RESULTS

We first considered the associations between usual drinking and each type of sexual behavior. Starting with low risk sex, the relationships between insertive and receptive oral sex and usual alcohol consumption were examined for each year, from 1985 through 1987. Ordinary least squares regression equations were used to predict the annual frequency of engaging in each type of oral sex from the measure of usual alcohol consumption. The unstandardized regression estimates and their standard errors are shown in Table 2. It can be seen that in wave 1 (1984-85) and wave 2 (1985-86) there was a significant direct association between the usual amount of alcohol consumed in a week and the frequency of both insertive and receptive oral sex; increased alcohol consumption predicted increased frequency of oral sex. However, this relationship was not significant in wave 3 (1986-87). During that year the association between oral sex and usual alcohol consumption diminished. The relationships shown in Table 2 were unaffected after statistically adjusting for lover status and age.

We next examined the relationships between high risk sex, (unprotected receptive and insertive anal intercourse), and usual alcohol consumption. Again, ordinary least squares regression models predicting the annual frequency of engaging in each type of unprotected intercourse from usual alcohol consumption were tested. These unstandardized regression coefficients and their standard errors are shown in Table 3. Unlike the results for oral sex, there was no significant association between either type of unprotected anal intercourse and drinking for any of the three annual time periods. The inclusion of age and lover status in the prediction models did not influence the results shown in Table 3.

Shifting now to the diagnostic indicator of alcohol abuse and dependence, we compared the group that met DIS/DSM-III criteria with the group that did not meet criteria on the four measures of sexual behavior. The means for each sexual behavior, broken down by alcoholism diagnosis, are shown for both wave 2 (1985-86) and wave 3 (1986-87) in Table 4. Log transformations were applied to the sexual behavior measures prior to conducting statistical tests for group mean differences. Looking first at 1985-86 results, it can be

Table 2

Unstandardized Ordinary Least Squares Regression Weights (SE)

Predicting Frequency of Oral Sex from Usual Alcohol Consumption

	Year		
Sexual behavior	1984-85	1985-86	1986-87
Receptive oral sex	.065**	.062**	.023
	(.02)	(.02)	(.02)
Insertive oral sex	.061**	.051**	.018
	(.02)	(.02)	(.02)

Note. Regression weights were estimated after adjusting for age
and lover status.

** p < .005

59

Table 3

Unstandardized Ordinary Least Squares Regression Weights (SE)

Predicting Unprotected Anal Intercourse from Usual Alcohol

Consumption

	Year		
Sexual behavior	1984-85	1985-86	1986-87
Unprotected receptive	.028	.017	-.003
anal intercourse	(.02)	(.01)	(.01)
Unprotected insertive	.031	.026	.004
anal intercourse	(.02)	(.02)	(.01)

Note. Regression weights were estimated after adjusting for age
and lover status.

Table 4

Frequency of Engaging in Four Sexual Behaviors Among Those Meeting DIS/DSM-

III Alcohol Abuse/Dependence Criteria Compared With Those Not Meeting

Criteria

	Year			
	1985-86		1986-87	
Sexual behavior	Dx. present	Dx. absent	Dx. present	Dx. absent
Receptive oral intercourse	38.4 (49.9)	41.4 (61.5)	55.7 (89.1)	34.8a (56.6)
Insertive oral intercourse	41.0 (59.4)	42.2 (60.6)	44.7 (79.9)	33.6 (54.1)
Unprotected receptive anal intercourse	7.3 (31.3)	7.0 (21.8)	5.0 (19.4)	5.7 (28.7)
Unprotected insertive anal intercourse	9.7 (33.8)	10.4 (29.2)	1.9 (6.0)	6.6 (23.5)

a $\underline{t}$ (602) = 1.96, $\underline{p} < .05$.

seen that there is no substantial or significant difference between the group diagnosed as alcoholic and those not diagnosed on the average annual frequency of engaging in the lower risk activities of receptive or insertive oral sex, or in the high risk activities of unprotected receptive or insertive anal intercourse. Both types of oral sex were performed approximately 40 times, on average, by both the alcoholic group and the non-alcoholic group. Both types of unprotected anal intercourse were performed approximately eight times, on average, by both groups.

Looking now at the 1986-87 results in Table 4, it can be seen that the alcoholic group reported one and a half times as many episodes of receptive oral sex compared with the non-alcoholic group; fifty-six compared with thirty-five, respectively. This difference was statistically significant. However, the differences between the two groups on insertive oral sex, and both types of unprotected anal intercourse were non-significant.

DISCUSSION

The findings presented here provide partial support for the general hypothesis that increased levels of alcohol consumption are associated with increased rates of sexual activity. This conclusion, however, is limited with respect to both the type of sexual behavior and the indicator of drinking. Sexual behaviors found to be related to drinking involved only receptive and insertive oral-genital sex; sexual activities considered by many to carry relatively low risk for transmission of HIV. The indicator of drinking which was most consistently related to these two sexual activities was usual weekly alcohol consumption. The DIS/DSM-III diagnostic indicator of alcohol abuse and dependence was more limited in its predictive power. The only significant difference between those diagnosed as alcoholic and those not diagnosed was the rate of receptive oral-genital sex. No difference between alcoholics and non-alcoholics was found for rates of insertive oral-genital sex.

The associations between the drinking measures and the measures of oral-genital sex must be interpreted cautiously since none of them were found consistently for all waves of data reported. The link between alcoholism and receptive oral sex was found only for the 1987 data but not for data collected in 1986. In contrast, the link between usual drinking and both type of oral sex was found for both 1985 and 1986 data, but disappeared in the 1987 data. The reasons for these alterations over time is unclear. However, the pattern of diminishing associations between usual drinking and oral sex parallels the pattern of associations between drug use and unprotected anal intercourse which was found in this panel sample in separate analyses (Martin, 1990b). While it is plausible that the link between drinking and oral sex is indeed becoming weaker over time in this sample, it must also be noted that the examination of these drinking data have been limited to repeated cross sectional analyses on the panel of gay men. Additional work involving longitudinal analyses is required before such an interpretation can be supported or refuted.

The lack of any significant associations between usual drinking or DIS/DSM-III alcoholism and unprotected anal intercourse fails to support the argument that drinking is associated with increased risk during sex. The lack of such a relationship for both receptive and insertive anal intercourse further suggests that drinking does not influence differentially the *taking* of risk compared with the *imposition* of risk during sex. The rates of neither of these activities appear to be heightened as a function of usual drinking patterns or alcoholism.

The discrepancy between the present findings and those reported by Stall and colleagues (Stall, 1988, 1989; Stall et al., 1986) is notable and should be resolved. While it is possible that the differences in findings represent true differences between the samples of gay men drawn from San Francisco and New York City, it is also possible that the differences are due to the measurement of sexual risk taking, i.e., the dependent variable, employed in each of these studies. In the present investigation we represented risk taking as specific and discreet sexual behaviors which vary not only in their biological risk of HIV transmission but also vary in their perceived degree of risk in the population. In contrast, the San Francisco group represented risk as a composite indicator ranging from no risk to high risk, which was composed of information on a number of specific sexual behaviors as well as partner characteristics (e.g., monogamy). The differences between Stall's representation of risk and the approach to representing risk taken by us may well explain the apparent differences in findings between the two studies.

An important limitation of the present findings is that the measures of drinking and alcoholism were not explicitly linked to sexual activity. That is, in the three waves of data reported here, we did not ask about the frequency of being under the influence of alcohol *during* episodes of sexual activity. Thus, conclusions drawn from these findings are limited with respect to the role played by alcohol in risk taking during sex. We may be able to address this question more directly in future analyses because we included questions about drinking during sex in interview data collected in 1988 and 1989. However, if the association between drinking and particular sexual behaviors is in fact diminishing over time, as the present findings suggest, we may have been too late in our attempt to remedy this shortcoming in the interview.

We should also note that the current analysis does not address the possibility that unusual or episodic periods of heavy drinking may result in increased sexual activity and increased risk taking during sex. While individuals who engaged in such episodes would tend to have higher scores on the measure of usual drinking, and they would also be more likely to meet DIS/DSM-III alcoholism criteria, we did not conduct analyses using an indicator of episodic heavy drinking. These data, however, are available and will be examined in future work.

In summary, this paper examined the association between relatively stable patterns of drinking and drinking problems and the frequency of engaging in high and low risk sexual behaviors in a broad community sample of gay men. Our findings suggest that drinking may be associated with increased rates of low risk sexual activity, i.e., receptive and insertive oral-genital sex, but not with increased rates of high risk sexual activity, i.e., unprotected anal intercourse. In addition, the findings also suggest that DIS/DSM-III alcoholism may be associated with a higher rate of receptive oral-genital sex. We failed to detect any differential relationship between the measure of usual drinking or alcoholism and either imposing risk on another by being the insertive partner during anal intercourse, or taking risk upon one's self by being the receptive partner during anal intercourse. Overall, the present findings cannot be taken as support for the hypothesis that alcohol is associated with high risk sexual behavior. However, before we can be confident with this conclusion for the present sample, further work on the question is clearly required. Such work must employ longitudinal analytic techniques which consider both the contemporaneous associations between alcohol and sexual behavior, as well as changes over time on these variables. Future work must also involve measures of drinking which focus on episodic bouts of intense alcohol consumption and sexual behavior occurring specifically while under the influence of alcohol.

REFERENCES

American Psychiatric Association. (1980). *Diagnostic and statistical manual of mental disorders (3rd Ed.)*. Washington, D.C.: Author.

Athanasiou, R., Shaver, P., & Tavris, C. (1970, July). Sex. *Psychology Today*, pp. 37-52.

Briddell, D. W., & Wilson, G. T. (1976). The effects of alcohol and expectancy set on male sexual arousal. *Journal of Abnormal Psychology*, *85*, 225-234.

Chmiel, J. S., Detels, R., Kaslow, R. A., Van Raden, M., Kingsley, L. A., & Brookmeyer, R. (1987). Factors associated with prevalent human immunodeficiency virus (HIV) infection in the Multicenter AIDS cohort study. *American Journal of Epidemiology*, *126*, 568-577.

Cooper, M. L., Skinner, J. B., George, W. H., & Brunner L. J. (1989, April). *Adolescent alcohol use and high risk sexual behaviors*. Paper presented at the Alcohol and AIDS Network Conference, Tucson, AZ.

Critchlow, B. (1983). Blaming the booze: The attribution of responsibility for drunken behavior. *Personality and Social Psychology Bulletin*, *9*, 451-473.

Critchlow, B. (1986). The powers of John Barleycorn: Beliefs about the effects of alcohol on social behavior. *American Psychologist*, *41*, 751-764.

Crowe, L. C., & George, W. H. (1989). Alcohol and human sexuality: Review and integration. *Psychological Bulletin*, *105*, 374-386.

Doll, L. (1989, April). *Alcohol use as a cofactor for disease and high-risk behavior*. Presented at the Alcohol and AIDS Network Conference, Tucson, AZ.

Hasin, D. S., & Grant, B. F. (1987). Assessment of specific drug disorders in a sample of substance abuse patients: A comparison of the DIS and the SADS-L procedures. *Drug and Alcohol Dependence*, *19*, 165-176.

Helzer, J. E., Robins, L. N., McEvoy, L. T., Spitznagle, E. L., Stoltzman, R. K., Farmer, A., & Brockington, I. F. (1985). A comparison of clinical and diagnostic interview schedule diagnoses. *Archives of General Psychiatry*, *42*, 657-666.

Jaffe, H. W., Choi, K., Thomas, P. D., et al. (1983). National case-control study of Kaposi's sarcoma and *Pneumocystis Carinii* pneumonia in homosexual men: Part 1, epidemiologic results. *Annals of Internal Medicine*, *99*(2), 145-151.

Kingsley, L. A., Kaslow, R., Rinaldo, C. R. Jr., Detre, K., Odaka, N., Van Raden, M., Detels, R., Polk, B. F., Chmiel, J., Kelsey, S. F., Ostrow, D., & Visscher, B. (1987). Risk factors for sero-conversion to human immunodeficiency virus among male homosexuals. *Lancet*, *1*, 345-349.

Leigh, B. C. (1989). In search of the seven dwarves: Issues of measurement and meaning in alcohol expectancy research. *Psychological Bulletin*, *105*, 361-373.

MacAndrew, C., & Edgerton, R. B. (1969). *Drunken comportment: A social explanation*. Chicago: Aldine.

Martin, J. L. (1987). The impact of AIDS on gay male sexual behavior patterns in New York City. *American Journal of Public Health*, *77*, 578-581.

Martin, J. L. (1990a). Drinking patterns and drinking problems in a community sample of gay men. In D. Seminara and A. Pawlowski (Eds.), *Alcohol, Immunomodulation and AIDS*, 27-34. New York: Alan R. Liss, Inc.

Martin, J. L. (1990b). Drug use and unprotected anal intercourse among gay men. *Health Psychology*, *9*, 450-465.

Martin, J. L., Dean, L., Garcia, M., & Hall, W. (1989). The impact of AIDS on a gay community: Changes in sexual behavior, substance use and mental health. *American Journal of Community Psychology*, *17*, 269-293.

Martin, J. L., Garcia, M. A., & Beatrice, S. (1989). Sexual behavior changes and HIV antibody in a cohort of New York City gay men. *American Journal of Public Health*, *79*, 501-503.

Mayer, K. H., Ayotte, D., Groopman, J. E., Stoddard, A., Sarngadharan, M., & Gallo, R. (1986). Association of human T-lymphotropic virus type III antibodies with sexual and other behaviors in a cohort of homosexual men from Boston with and without generalized lymphadenopathy. *American Journal of Medicine*, *80*, 357-363.

Moss, A. R., Osmond, D., Bacchetti, P., Chermann, J. C., Barre-Sinoussi, F., & Carlson, J. (1987). Risk factors for AIDS and HIV seropositivity in homosexual men. *American Journal of Epidemiology*, *125*, 1035-1047.

Polk, B. F., Fox, R., Brookmeyer, R., Kanchanaraksa, S., Kaslow, R., Visscher, B., Rinaldo, C., & Phair, J. (1987). Predictors of the acquired immunodeficiency syndrome developing in a cohort of seropositive homosexual men. *New England Journal of Medicine*, *316*, 63-66.

Robins, L. N., Helzer, J. E., Weissman, M. M., Orvashel, H., Gruenberg, E., Burke, J. D., & Regier, D. A. (1984). Lifetime prevalence of specific psychiatric disorders in three sites. *Archives of General Psychiatry*, *41*, 942-948.

Robins, L. N., Helzer, J. E., Ratcliff, K. S., & Seyfried, W. (1982). Validity of the diagnostic interview schedule, version II: DSM-III diagnoses. *Psychological Medicine*, *12*, 855-870.

Rockwell, K., Ellinwood, E., & Kantor, C. (1973). Drugs and sex: Scene of ambivalence. *Journal of the American College Health Association*, *21*, 483-488.

Room, R., & Collins, G. Eds.).(1983). *Drinking and disinhibition: Nature and meaning of the link* (NIAAA Monograph No. 12). Washington, D.C.: U.S. Government Printing Office.

Stall, R., McKusick, L., Wiley, J., Coates, T. J., & Ostrow, D. G. (1986). Alcohol and drug use during sexual activity and compliance with safe sex guidelines for AIDS: The AIDS behavioral research project. *Health Education Quarterly, 13*, 359-371.

Stall, R. (1988). The prevention of HIV infection associated with drug and alcohol use during sexual activity. *Advances in Alcohol and Substance Abuse, #7*, 73-88.

Stall, R. (1989, April). *A combination of alcohol and drug use, and high risk factors for HIV infection.* Paper presented at the Alcohol and AIDS Network Conference, Tucson, AZ.

Stevens, C. E., Taylor, P. E., Zang, E. A., Morrison, J. M., Harley, E. J., de Cordoba, S. R., Bacino, C., Ting, R. C. Y., Bodner, A. J., Sarngadharan, M. G., Gallo, R. C., & Rubinstein, P. (1986). Human T-cell lymphotropic virus type III infection in a cohort of homosexual men in New York City. *Journal of the American Medical Association, 265*(16), 2267-2272.

Turner, C. F., Miller, H. E., & Moses, L. E. (1989). *AIDS, Sexual Behavior and Intravenous Drug Use.* Washington, D.C.: National Academy Press.

Winkelstein, W. Jr., Lyman, D. M., & Padian, N. S. (1987). Sexual practices and risk of infection by the AIDS-associated retrovirus: The San Francisco Men's Health Study. *Journal of the American Medical Association, 257*, 321-325.

Shooting Galleries, Their Proprietors, and Implications for Prevention of AIDS

J. Bryan Page, PhD
Prince C. Smith, MHA
Normie Kane

SUMMARY. Locales where intravenous drug users (IVDUs) go to inject themselves are of special interest, in preventing the spread of AIDS. Field research conducted among IVDUs in Miami, Florida answers questions about opportunities for infection in shooting galleries and outlines the cultural context in which risky injection occurs. Intervention among proprietors of shooting galleries has potential for successful prevention of infection, but success may only be short-term without ongoing reinforcement of prevention techniques.

INTRODUCTION

Locales where intravenous drug users (hereafter, IVDUs) go to inject themselves are of special interest in preventing the spread of AIDS. Several researchers, including Marmor et al. (1987), and Drucker (1986) have indicated that safe houses, often called "shooting galleries" in the literature on drug abuse, provide multiple opportunities for exposure to the human immunodeficiency virus (hereafter, HIV) through interchange of blood traces in used syringes and needles. Blood-to-blood or body fluid-to-blood contact is necessary for passing the HIV from one person to another, and the practice of "booting" (drawing blood into the syringe before injecting the drug) makes blood available in the syringe for

---

J. Bryan Page, Prince C. Smith, and Normie Kane are affiliated with the University of Miami, School of Medicine, Department of Psychiatry.

contact with the circulatory system of another IVDU, depending on how well the previous user has cleaned the syringe. Shooting galleries vary widely in their handling of IVDUs and their paraphernalia, but they are generally assumed to proliferate infective contacts among IVDUs through the common use of syringes and needles that are contaminated with the blood of other IVDUs. The present paper examines some aspects of behavior in shooting galleries that offer opportunities for preventing the spread of HIV in this population.

BACKGROUND

Intravenous drug use in shooting galleries has been identified as especially risky for HIV infection since at least, 1985 (cf. Centers for Disease Control, 1989; Des Jarlais, Friedman, & Hopkins, 1985; Ginzberg, Weiss, McDonald & Hubbard, 1985). Most scholarly accounts of these phenomena are written at considerable distance from human behavior that they describe and analyze. The first perspective on the relationship between AIDS and intravenous drug use came from retrospective data gathered from people with active cases of AIDS (cf. Maayan, Wormser, & Hewlett, 1985). The need for more information about the epidemic led to studies of captive IVDU populations in centers for treatment of drug abuse (cf. Friedland et al., 1985; Robertson et al., 1986). Larger epidemiologic studies of non-captive populations (cf. Des Jarlais, Friedman, & Hopkins, 1985) and mixed populations recruited from treatment centers and the street (Chaisson, Moss, Onishi, Osmond & Carlton, 1987; Des Jarlais, Friedman & Hopkins, 1985) yielded a still broader perspective on how people become infected with the HIV. In this gradual broadening of perspective, all of the treatments of shooting behavior are written in general aggregate terms, based on self-reports of IVDUs who volunteer to divulge information on their personal drug use to interviewers.

These studies have taught us that IVDUs engage in several kinds of behavior that place them at risk of exposure (blood-to-blood contact) to the HIV. Sharing of needles (Marmor et al., 1987; Drucker, 1986; Wolk et al., 1988) is one such behavior, as is use of the same "cooker," the receptacle in which water and powdered drugs are mixed (Marmor et al., 1987). Another risky behavior described in the literature is the use of hypodermic apparatus (hereafter, "works") rented from the shooting gallery (Des Jarlais, Friedman & Hopkins, 1985). These behaviors all appear to be elicitable from the IVDUs in aggregate, but the literature does not give a sense of how they fit together into a pattern of behavior among the users.

Important questions remain unanswered by these treatments of the relationship between intravenous drug use and infection by the HIV. For example, in this age of cheap, disposable hypodermic syringes, why would IVDUs share works? Also, there exists a belief among IVDUs that an injection of the wrong blood type leads to an unpleasant experience called a "bone-crusher." Why, in light of this belief, would IVDUs not clean works before sharing them? Finally, because the shooting galleries have always had a bad reputation for cleanliness, why would IVDUs continue to resort to them in the face of the AIDS epidemic?

To answer these questions, it is necessary first to look to the existing literature on the subculture among IVDUs. Ethnographic literature on IV drug use and the lifestyles of users tends to be at least fifteen years old (cf. Agar, 1973; Preble & Casey, 1969). At that time, works were illegal in many states and disposable works were not widely available. The accounts of injection (hereafter, "shooting") behavior described sharing of a single set of works primarily because of scarcity and illegality (Agar, 1973, p. 65). There was precedent for sharing of works in the ethnographic literature, but it did not help to explain the continued sharing behavior thought to persist among present-day IVDUs. The ethnographic literature does not mention cleaning syringes with water. Because water at room temperature does not kill the virus, the answer to the question about cleaning may be that IVDUs have practiced cleaning, but the rinsing with water was ineffective in stopping the virus.

Perhaps most instructive of the ethnographic contributions to understanding of present-day patterns of IV drug use is the institution of the shooting gallery. Many users do not have sufficient control of their living environments to be able to inject themselves regularly at home. Since injecting oneself on the street risks arrest and other forms of social opprobrium, the shooting gallery (or "get-off" as it is called in Miami) offers an attractive alternative for this kind of

IVDU, where he or she can go and inject drugs in the company of people who tolerate this behavior. In the absence of a more comfortable place in which to shoot, the IVDU is likely to opt for the get-off.

The available literature affords at least three hypotheses for testing through an update of the ethnography of drug injection:

1. Sharing of works is related to continued observance of ritualistic drug sharing among IVDUs.
2. Although cleaning of works has been common among IVDUs, the cleaning methods are ineffective against the HIV.
3. Shooting galleries continue to draw clientele who have no other locale where they can shoot up.

In addition to these hypotheses, the present investigation should also be able to:

1. describe additional behaviors taking place in get-offs that place the clientele at risk of infection by the HIV.
2. develop an understanding of the present cultural context in which risky behavior persists, and
3. suggest strategies for intervening at key points in the behavior of IVDUs in get-offs for the prevention of further spread of HIV infection..

This paper will use ethnographic data gathered in a street-based ethnographic study to test these hypotheses and provide these descriptions and suggestions.

METHODS

The study reported in this paper focuses on the population least likely to be captured in studies of IVDUs in clinical settings, a street-recruited group of IVDUs. Networks of informal social relations are the principal tools of the research team attempting to identify illegal drug users, because large-scale probability sampling is inefficient in identifying sufficiently large numbers of people engaged in a relatively rare behavior. Several studies (Carter, Coggins, & Doughty, 1980; Chitwood & Morningstar, 1985; Page,

McKay, Rio & Sweeney, 1983) have used network tracing methods successfully in studies with substantial ethnographic components. The present study built series of contacts in neighborhoods known for activity in intravenous drug use into a total of 233 contacts ascertained to be IVDUs.

To make this number of contacts, the field team had to screen 521 individuals who were presented as IVDUs who had not been in treatment for at least six months. Of the 233 individuals who passed the screening criteria, two were determined to be participants in treatment and were placed in a parallel study of IVDUs in treatment. One individual managed to gain acceptance in both the treatment and street study, as well as a clinical study at the local Veterans Administration hospital. His responses to the interviews in the three studies were so discordant that he was ejected from all studies. The group of 230 study participants provided several varieties of data to the street project:

Blood Tests

To determine seroprevalence in the baseline population and incidence of seroconversion in a longitudinal study, the study participants gave blood samples which were tested for presence of HIV antibodies by an enzyme-linked immunosorbent assay (ELISA) technique. In cases of first-time seropositivity, the samples were retested with the ELISA method, and, if still positive, were confirmed by a Western Blot technique. In addition to the seroassays, the study subjects' blood samples also underwent a series of descriptive and functional studies of the peripheral immune system. The field team conducted repetitions of these tests at six-month intervals after baseline.

Interview Schedule

Basic sociodemographic and risk behavior data were elicited from the 230 study participants in an interview conducted at the time of the baseline. The risk assessment items concentrated on drug injection behavior and sexual behavior, and it covered a period roughly ten years prior to the baseline interview, divided into segments five, four, and one year in duration (ten years to five years before the interview, five years to one year before the interview, and the year immediately before the interview). A repetition of risk behavior and medical history over the last six months is repeated at six-month intervals during the longitudinal study of these participants.

Needle Use Values Interview

To understand and update the cultural background and underlying motivations for using syringes to ingest drugs, the field team has conducted in-depth, open-ended interviews with a subset of the study population. The format of the tape-recorded interview allows the respondent to structure a narrative about his/her relationship with the needle according to his/her own perceptions. The tapes are transcribed verbatim and coded for content retrievability, using a version of the Outline of Cultural Materials (Murdock et al., 1961). The field team has conducted 33 interviews and coded 20 transcriptions.

Direct Observation of Needle Using Behavior

Focused observation on the use of injection apparatus in natural habitats is a unique feature of the present study. The field team has conducted fifteen observational sessions in which 53 IVDUs participated. Field workers enter locales where shooting takes place and observe use and care of needles. If study participants are injecting drugs at the time of the observation, a brief protocol is filled out for each of the participants. Field notes in narrative form are also part of the data gathered in this anthropological phase of the study.

Network Characteristics of the Study Population

Field workers gather data on the informal social relations among study participants. The field team includes in observational notes occasions when people are seen to inject drugs together and/or to hang out together. People who present together at the blood test center are also noted, as are shooting and sexual partners identified in risk interviews.

The data described above are still being collected, and final analysis of longitudinal data is still months away. Other publications present results of interview schedule responses and blood tests (Page, Morgan, Chitwood & Smith). The analysis of the needle use values interviews is also incomplete. Nevertheless, the current analysis of all of the project's data informs the work presented here. Observational materials analyzed to date provide the bulk of the data in the present paper.

RESULTS

At baseline, 47 percent (106 of 230) of the study participants were seropositive for antibodies to the HIV. Fifteen are known to have died of AIDS to date, but most seropositive participants remain asymptomatic. Numbers of shots taken during the ten years prior to the baseline interview is related to seropositivity, $t(228) = -3.84, p < .001$ on a univariate basis (Page & Chitwood, 1988), while use of get-off houses during the period five years to one year before the baseline interview contributes substantially to a logistic regression multivariate model of risk behavior in prediction of baseline seropositivity (Page, Morgan, Chitwood & Smith). These results continue to focus attention on what happens in the shooting gallery that makes it so risky for HIV infection.

Observations of behavior in get-offs in Miami can be used to redefine the areas of risk in patronizing these establishments. The field team has conducted fifteen observational sessions in a total of nine different get-offs. These places are variable in their management and atmosphere, ranging from a very business-like establishment, with a formal entry fee paid to a house man at the door, to a single room run by a lone individual who will exchange the use of his/her room for a share of the drugs to be consumed by the client. In all but two of these establishments, there were no new, packaged, disposable syringes in evidence. Shooting sessions may take place in groups or individually, with needles provided by the house (sometimes for a fee, sometimes included as a house courtesy to the customer paying an entry fee). These needles are stored in a common container, usually either a coffee can or a cloth pouch. The house almost always has enough works to allow everyone in the group to shoot at once. In fact, in the fifteen sessions observed, during which no fewer than 150 injections have taken place, the field team has yet to observe a clear case of needle sharing between two IVDUs.

Therein lies the answer to the first question posed in the background section of this paper: in most situations, IVDUs do not share needles at all. They draw needles from pools of used needles maintained by the shooting gallery. This, as we shall see later, is tantamount to inadvertent sharing with possibly unknown partners who used the works before the present shooter. In answer to the second question about cleaning of needles between injections, our observations have found that IVDUs usually clean needles loaned by the house, because the house requires it. The small, diabetic-gauge disposable syringes and needles preferred by IVDUs inevitably become clogged and inoperable after repeated injections. To forestall this condition, the house rules in all houses observed in Miami dictate that after each use of a set of works, the customer must clean the set with "dirty water" (water provided for cleaning purposes) before returning the syringe and needle to the storage container. Every needle returned to the container is supposed to be returned after this kind of "cleaning." A spot-testing of needles collected from storage cans and pouches of several local get-offs in Miami yielded an ELISA seropositivity rate of testable syringes and needles of ten percent (Chitwood et al., 1990). Given the high frequency of use among many of the study participants, regular patronage of a get-off house should lead to regular exposure to HIV-antibody-seropositive syringes and needles.

There are other aspects of patronizing get-off houses that place their clientele at risk of exposure to HIV. One example of this risk is the use of "clean water" by multiple clients. Clean water is the name given to the small container (often a baby food jar) from which water is drawn to be mixed with drugs. As most Miamian drug injection behavior involves cocaine, which is not "cooked" during the mixing process, whatever microbes are in the clean water will be injected into the shooter. Even if the client uses a new set of works to inject the drug, the water mixed with the drugs could be contaminated by exposure to contaminated syringes. As of this writing, the research team has not yet tested this water, but we plan to do so in the near future.

The manner of sharing drugs observed in some get-off houses

also carries possibilities of intercontamination of drug doses. People who intend to share quantities of speedball must mix the cocaine and heroin in separate caps to avoid heating the cocaine. They may then draw the cocaine into one syringe and the heroin into another, squirting the heroin into the cocaine syringe through its nozzle and squirting half of the mixture, called speedball, back into the syringe that originally contained heroin. If either syringe contains virus at the start of such an operation, both are likely to contain it after it is finished. Squirting drugs from one syringe to another also has taken place among larger groups observed by the field team.

In addition to these regularly occurring risks of exposure in Miami's get-off houses, there are some minor risks involving accidental punctures by contaminated needles. Get-offs tend to be crowded and poorly lit, with several people injecting at more or less the same time. If a shooter loses the vein into which he or she is trying to inject drugs, he or she may spend several minutes trying to find another vein. During this time, the syringe may be held loosely in the hand or even put down on a bed or chair. As yet, the field team has not observed an accidental puncture, but the possibilities are extensive in the environment of the shooting gallery.

Lifestyles of people who inject drugs are variable, but the field research team in Miami has encountered numerous cases of individuals whose living arrangements do not allow them to shoot up in their own residences. Single men who live with their families of orientation must find habitats outside of the home for most of their shooting activity. This is also true for married men whose spouses do not permit shooting in their own homes. Other individuals who live in domiciliary facilities or boarding houses may not have safe places for self-injection outside of the get-off house. We have observed that shooting galleries in Miami do not lack clientele, even though there appears to be a general understanding among IVDUs that the risk of infection by the HIV is great in these places.

As mentioned earlier, management of shooting galleries observed by the field team varies from formal to informal, but there is usually one person who assures adherence to house rules. The following description of action in a get-off house in Miami summarizes field notes taken at one place during the course of four observational visits spaced over eleven months.

Time 1, June, 1988 — We arrive at subject # 4367's apartment, and his mother greets us at the door. My guide explains to me that she is the recipient of the house fee, because we are in her apartment, so I pay the woman $10 for the priviledge of entering the apartment. 4367 emerges from the bathroom and ushers us into a back bedroom where three men are seated on crates and chairs. He directs us to sit on the bed. He reaches behind the bed and pulls out a pouch from which he produces four syringes, one for 4367, one for my guide, and two for the men already there. The third man has brought his own gimmick (syringe and needle) with him. The participants, including my guide all have their own drugs, having recently purchased nickel bags before coming to 4367's place. 4367 places two jars of water, one a large peanut butter jar and the other a baby food jar. The larger jar is designated dirty water and the smaller, clean water. The three men who were already in the room have decided to make speedball, because they have both "boy" (heroin) and "girl" (cocaine). Using separate twist-off aluminum bottle caps with the plastic liners removed, two of them mix drugs with water drawn from the baby food jar, the heroin cap being brought to a boil with a lit half-book of matches. The drugs are then drawn into separate syringes. One of the speedball sharing group removes the needle from his syringe and allows the contents of the other syringe to be squirted into his syringe from the other one. He then replaces his needle and squirts the mixture into the other two men's syringes. 4367 reminds them that they need to "take care" of him, and each obliges by squirting a small portion from their works into 4367's works, amid complaints about their stinginess and ingratitude. All four inject themselves with the speedball mixture, booting once. They then set about cleaning their works by drawing water through the needle and "skeeting" (squirting) that water into a piece of tissue paper held in the palm of the hand. Wet tissues are thrown into a wastebasket. The group repeats the operation, always drawing from the jar containing dirty water, until the water in the syringes appears clear. 4367 talks almost continuously throughout the session, repeating instructions on which water jar is which, how the works must be cleaned after use, and admonitions to keep squirting until the water in the syringe is clear. My guide also twists a piece of tissue and removes the plunger from his syringe, using the twisted paper to swab out the neck of the syringe. The participants return the syringes to 4367's bag before leaving.

Time 2, September, 1988--My guide and I arrive at 4367's house and find his mother sitting on a bed by the back door where I pay our entry fee. She yells to 4367 that we have arrived, and he emerges from the bathroom a few minutes later with another man whom I do not know. Another man enters the apartment a few minutes later, and 4367 shows us to the back bedroom, which now has a large pile of clothes stacked in one corner. He places two brown bottles on a small table in the middle of the room. Both are somewhat less than half full of chlorine bleach. The five people sit around the room on crates and small chairs and the double bed. 4367 produces four sets of works from his pouch and passes them to the four participants. All of the participants are familiar faces. One is my guide, who is an old friend of 4367, and the other two participated in the last observed shooting session. Cocaine is the only drug used in this session, and it is mixed in separate caps, representing the drugs contributed by two different parties. 4367 exacts his share in the usual way, having drugs squirted into his works from another syringe. One of the participants has trouble getting blood to pay back into his syringe, so my guide volunteers to be a "doctor" and find a proper vein into which to inject the cocaine. He has to work several different zones, but he eventually finds a vein on the other man's lower forearm that pays back blood, indicating a successful "hit" on a vein. When all have completed their injections, 4367 points at the bleach and directs them to use that before using the dirty water. All participants draw and squirt the chlorine bleach from the small brown bottles at least twice before using the dirty water. My guide and one other participant also swab the barrels of their works with paper before returning them to 4367.

Time 3, February, 1989—I arrive with a co-field worker and guide, and we are told that 4367 is in the bathroom. We sit in the living room and talk with other family members and guests while we wait for 4367. He emerges and asks if we have taken care of his mother. She is in the other room, and I pay her our fee when I find her there. Among the guests today are one person who was present at *Time 1*, one who is in the study but has not been seen previously at this get-off, and a new person to whom we are introduced. During the conversation, we find that two of the guests are veterans. 4367 ushers us into the back bedroom, which he hastily arranges into a circle of chairs and crates at the bedside to accomodate the seven people in the group. He passes syringes taken from his pouch to the five people who intend to shoot drugs in this session. My guide has not brought any with him, and he asks if anyone else would like for him to cop for them. Everyone else has drugs, so he leaves to buy a nickel bag. While he is gone, 4367 talks about some of the styles of shooting practiced by other regular clients of his house. He says that one man will not allow anyone to leave the room until his cocaine high has subsided. When my guide returns, the guests begin mixing the cocaine with water from the baby food jar. They draw drugs from the caps without interchanging between syringes, and 4367 takes his share directly from the two caps, complaining at how little was left for him. He says that he treats his guests right, but they just won't treat him right. When the shooting is over (all guests hit themselves efficiently) the cleaning process begins, and my guide asks if there is any chlorine. 4367 replies that he ran out, but he has a small bottle of alcohol that should be alright. He brings that bottle in from another room and places it on the table. He tells the guests that they can use it if they want. Some, including the guide, squirt two charges of alcohol through the works before using the dirty water. Two do not, using only the dirty water. All return their works to 4367's pouch.

Time 4, May, 1989 — I arrive with a guide, another study participant, and a field worker during a rainstorm when 4367's apartment is especially crowded. His mother is not in, so I pay the entry fee to his sister. Again, 4367 is in the bathroom, and he takes about 20 minutes to emerge. The crowd in the living room includes small children, shooters, adult siblings of 4367, and friends of those siblings. 4367 emerges from the bathroom with two shooters, both participants in the study. They leave, and we go into the bedroom to wait for one of my companions, who has gone to purchase drugs with money collected from other participants. He returns in fifteen minutes, and four of us sit in the back bedroom at the foot of the bed. 4367 passes works from a cigar box pulled from a drawer. Clean and dirty water are in very small containers on top of a dresser at that end of the room. There is no evidence of any chlorine bleach or alcohol in the room. The men mix the drugs into a single cap and draw their shares from the same cap, amid 4367's complaints that nobody leaves any for him. Each is efficient in finding and shooting into a vein. They each clean their works with the dirty water, taking care to swab out the barrel with tissue. They then return the works to 4367's cigar box when they finish cleaning them.

DISCUSSION

The preceding descriptive accounts and four brief narratives afford an opportunity to highlight parts of the physical process of injecting drugs and the social setting in which this is done for purposes of preventing the spread of HIV infection. In the course of preparing to inject drugs, we have seen several junctures at which additional chance of exposure occurs. The communal use of clean water for drug mixing probably adds somewhat to the risk of infection, as does sharing of caps. Maintaining separate jars of water for each user that are changed after each session and sufficient caps so that each user has his or her own might reduce these kinds of risks somewhat. Nevertheless, it is easier to measure out mixed drugs than to measure out equal amounts of powdered drugs when dividing a shared dose. It is easier to calibrate equity along the barrel of a syringe than in the bottom of a cap. Separate caps may precipitate more disputes over fair sharing. If all participants in a shooting session were using new syringes for each injection, sharing from syringe to syringe might be less risky.

Dangers related to crowded conditions in the get-offs will be difficult to control, although 4367's sessional style could be useful in avoiding accidents. People do not enter and leave easily during one of 4367's sessions, and there is not much movement of people around drug-and-blood-laden works during a given session. He chooses room size according to the size of the group (the bathroom for one or two people, the bedroom for groups of up to ten) and allows entry and exit reluctantly.

The most important aspect of 4367's management of his get-off house is his enforcement of house rules. During the summer of, 1988, some of his clients were randomized into the intensive intervention of a project to reduce risk of HIV infection among IVDUs. The addition of project-issued bleach bottles to his shooting equipment was noticeable at the *Time 2* session, but the apparent influence of the clients participating in the intervention appeared to wear off by *Time 3* and all but disappear by *Time 4*. Still, he continues to exercise control over how shooting proceeds among his clients throughout each of the sessions. An intervention that included 4367 could take full advantage of his ability to control proceedings in his get-off, and it would have wide influence in reducing injection-related risk in the IVDU population in 4367's neighborhood.

The idea of intervention among proprietors of shooting galleries is not new. ADAPT, a community-based organization of ex-IVDUs who have been working in the area of New York City to prevent HIV infection among active IVDUs, have been supplying bleach and alcohol to managers of shooting galleries for several years (Goldsmith, 1987). The reports on participation by proprietors of shooting galleries were generally positive, and the rationale for that kind of intervention was straightforward. Shooting galleries whose clients all die of AIDS soon will have no customers left.

It was evident in the observation of 4367's get-off that the immediate impact of the brief (three sessions) intervention in which he participated was positive. The intervention lacked sustaining power in modifying his behavior, however, and it failed to institute cleaning of works both before and after use. If 4367 had been consistent in requiring chlorine rinses after each use of his works, that in itself may have been effective in preventing contagion within his clientele. Cleaning before and after is the recommended technique for general needle use, because a shooter cannot assume that the needle he or she is about to use has been cleaned properly by the previous shooter. An improved intervention that reinforced at regular intervals the prevention techniques learned by 4367 and insured that those techniques took a more generally applicable form (i.e., cleaning both before and after use of needles, rather than simply cleaning after) could have a major impact among IVDUs served by 4367's get-off.

The present study's field team has encountered some sentiment among proprietors of shooting galleries in Miami that they are interested in keeping their clientele alive and free of AIDS. One manager of two different get-offs has spontaneously instituted a policy of new needles only in his houses. He is not part of the study population, and in fact had instituted his policy before meeting members of the field team. His houses are relatively clean, and they are the only places visited by the field team where new works in packages were available. In one establishment, the works were in a basket hung in a macrame sling in the living room. No used needles were present intact. This proprietor claimed that he required works to be broken and discarded after use. In the other house run by this individual, the needles were also said to be new, but only half were still in wrappers. Additional amenities in this establishment included saline solution for mixing with drugs and a separate room for smoking crack. Because observations have just begun in these establishments, it remains to be seen whether the new needle policy represents a lasting commitment on the part of this proprietor. Nevertheless, he has several times expressed his desire to keep his clientele alive, because his livelihood depends on their coming back to his houses. To varying degrees, most of the proprietors contacted to date would agree with the logic of the proprietor who advocates new needles only. The conduct of 4367 indicates, however, that prevention efforts cannot rely on a single conversion experience to have a lasting impact on proprietors of shooting galleries. They will need ongoing encouragement to maintain non-contagious shooting practices in the houses for which they are responsible.

REFERENCES

Agar, M. H. (1973). *Ripping and Running*, New York: Academic Press.

Carter, W. E., Coggins, W. J. & Doughty, P. L. (1980). *Cannabis in Costa Rica*. Philadelphia: ISHI Press.

Centers for Disease Control (1989). Update: Acquired Immunodeficiency Syndrome – United States, 1981-1988. *Mortality and Morbidity Weekly Report 38* (14), 230-249.

Chaisson, R. E., Moss, A. R., Onishi, R., Osmond, D., & Carlson, J. R. (1987). Human immunodeficiency virus infection in heterosexual intravenous drug users in San Francisco. *American Journal of Public Health*, 77(2), 169-171.

Chitwood, D. D., McCoy, C. B., Fletcher, M. A., Page, J. B., Inciardi, J. A., McBride, D. C., Comerford, M., Trapido, E., & McCoy, V. (1989). HIV seropositivity rates among needles from "shooting galleries" in Miami, Florida. *American Journal of Public Health* (in press).
Chitwood, D. D., & Morningstar, P. C. (1985). Factors which differentiate cocaine users in treatment from non-treatment users. *The International Journal of the Addictions*, *20*(3), 453-463.
Des Jarlais, D. C., Friedman, S. R., & Hopkins, W. (1985). Risk reduction for the acquired immunodeficiency syndrome among intravenous drug users. *Annals of Internal Medicine 103*, 755-759.Drucker, E. (1986). Aids and addiction in New York City. *American Journal of Drug and Alcohol Abuse*, *12*(1&2), 165-181.
Friedland G. H., Harris, C., Butkus-Small, C., Shine, D., Moll B., Darrow, W., & Klien, R. (1985). Intravenous drug abusers and the acquired immunodeficiency syndrome (AIDS): demographic, drug use, and needle-sharing patterns. *Archives of Internal Medicine 8*: 1413-1437.
Friedman, S. R., Des Jarlais, D. C., Kleinman, P., Sotheran, J. L., Marmor, M., & Mauge, C. (1988). Risk reduction among intravenous drug users in and out of treatment. *Abstracts of presentations at the IV International Conference on AIDS, Stockholm, Sweden. Abstract # 8013*, 452.
Ginzburg, H., Weiss, S. H., MacDonald, M. G., & Hubbard, R. L. (1985). HTLV-III exposure among drug users. *Cancer Research Supplement*, *45*, 46055-46085.
Goldsmith, D. (1987). *AIDS risk reduction education for IV drug users in New York City*. Paper presented at the annual meetings of the Society for Applied Anthropology, Oaxaca, Mexico.
Maayan, S., Wormser, G. P., & Hewlett, D. (1985). Acquired immunodeficiency syndrome (AIDS) in an economically disadvantaged population. *Archives of Internal Medicine*, *45*:1607-1612.
Marmor, M., Des Jarlais, D. C., Cohen, H., Friedman, S. R., Beatrice, S. Dubin, N., El-Sadr, W., Mildvan, D., Yancovitz, S., Mathur, U., & Holzman, R. (1987). Risk factors for infection with human immunodeficiency virus among intravenous drug abusers in New York City. *AIDS 1*(1), 39-44.
Morningstar, P. C., & Chitwood, D. D. (1984). Cocaine users' view of themselves: implicit personality theory in context. *Human Organization 43*(2), 307-318.
Murdock, G. P., Ford, C. S., Hudson, A. E., Kennedy, R., Simmons, L.W., & Whiting, J. W. M. (1961). Outline of Cultural Materials. *New Haven: Human Relations Area Files, Inc.*
Page, J. B., McKay, C., Rio, L., & Sweeney, J. (1983). *Ethnography of prescription drug use among women in Dade County, Florida*. (Grant # 1 RO1 DA 02675). Rockville, Maryland: National Institute on Drug Abuse.
Page, J. B., Morgan, R., Chitwood, D. D., & Smith, P. C. Predicting HIV-1 seropositivity among active IV drug users. Manuscript submitted for publication.

Page, J. B., & Chitwood, D. D. (1988). Seropositivity among street-recruited IV drug users. *Abstracts of presentations at the IV International Conference on AIDS, Stockholm, Sweden. Abstract # 8005*, 450.

Preble, E., & Casey, J. J. (1969). Taking care of business: the heroin user's life on the street. *International Journal of the Addictions*, 4(1), 1-24.

Robertson J. R., Bucknall, A. B. V., Welsby, P. D., Roberts, J. J. K., Inglis, J. M., Peutherer, J. F., & Brettle, R. P. (1986). Epidemic of AIDS related virus (HTLV-III/LAV) infection among intravenous drug abusers. *British Medical Journal*, *292*, 5-12.

Wiedman, D. D., & Page, J. B. (1982). Drug use on the street and on the beach: Cubans and Anglos in Miami, Florida. *Urban Anthropology*, *11*(2), 212-226.

Wolk, J., Wodak, A., Morlet, A., Guinan, J., Wilson, E., Gold, J., & Cooper, D. A. (1988). Syringe HIV seroprevalence and behavioural and demographic characteristics of intravenous drug users in Sydney, Australia. *AIDS*, *2*, 373-377.

AIDS Prevention with Drug Users: Health Psychology Research

James L. Sorensen, PhD

SUMMARY. This article provides an overview of AIDS prevention with intravenous drug users. It is vital to prevent the spread of HIV among intravenous drug users and to slow the spread from them to their sexual partners and future progeny. The conceptual models of health psychology can help planners to understand the background and design the interventions that are needed, but these models do not fit perfectly to the problems associated with AIDS. The development of one line of AIDS prevention research is described, involving group and individual education of intravenous drug abusers and their sexual partners. The problem of AIDS among drug abusers provides an opportunity for health psychologists to apply their craft to an area of national importance.

Imagine that the President of the United States created a position of "Psychologist General" similar to the position of Surgeon General in the executive branch of government. What would the Psychologist General recommend to prevent the spread of AIDS? With some knowledge of health psychology, the Psychologist General's

James L. Sorensen is affiliated with the Department of Psychiatry and the Center for AIDS Prevention Studies, University of California, San Francisco.

Reprint requests should be sent to the author at Substance Abuse Services — Ward 92, UCSF at San Francisco General Hospital, 1001 Potrero Avenue, San Francisco, CA 94110.

An earlier version of this paper was presented at the University of California intercampus conference entitled "Health Psychology Research on AIDS," June 23-25, 1988, Berkeley, CA. This work was supported by NIMH/NIDA grant number MH42459 and NIDA grant number DA04340. The author appreciates the cooperation of the staff and patients of substance abuse services, UCSF at San Francisco General Hospital, and the AIDS prevention efforts of Les Pappas and the San Francisco AIDS Foundation.

87

recommendations might include the following: (1) Information and fear of AIDS do not create behavior change, but they may be precursors to changing the activities that put people at risk; (2) we must teach people what to do, not just what to avoid, and repeatedly deliver the message through multiple channels of communication; (3) to be effective with the people most at risk, AIDS prevention techniques must take into account the values of these different groups. These principles would be particularly apt in preventing the spread of HIV among intravenous drug users.

This paper describes the issues of AIDS prevention with intravenous drug users, a group among whom AIDS prevention is vital to our national interests.

INTRAVENOUS DRUG USE AND AIDS

Epidemiological surveillance of AIDS and HIV infection reveals that intravenous drug users are a continued and growing group at risk. For the last several years intravenous drug users have comprised about 25% of the cases of AIDS (Centers for Disease Control [CDC], 1987). The 1988 statistics reveal that drug users accounted for 30% of the cases in that year (CDC, 1988). Ethnic minorities are overrepresented with regard to their frequency in the population among AIDS cases, as has been well documented (Bakeman, McCray, Lumb, Jackson, & Whitley, 1987). It is important to recognize that just as minority issues are important in understanding AIDS, drug abuser issues are important in understanding minority AIDS: Of the Caucasian men with AIDS only 12% are intravenous drug users. Of Black and Hispanic men, however, 40% acquired AIDS through the needle. These racial differences are even more pronounced among women and pediatric cases of AIDS. Regional differences in AIDS incidence indicate that 80% of the intravenous drug user AIDS cases have been in the Northeast. Information on rates of infection indicates similarly that in some areas of the Northeastern United States most intravenous drug users have been infected with HIV. But in most other areas of the country the vast majority of intravenous drug users have not yet been infected with the AIDS virus. If prevention techniques are developed which are effective, and if these techniques are effectively disseminated to intravenous drug users in the Midwest, South, and West, then AIDS prevention with drug users can be an achievable objective.

There are clear behavioral connections between AIDS and intravenous drug use; the evidence is not just epidemiological. Faltz and Madover (1987) point to five connections between substance abuse and AIDS:

1. direct transmission (sharing blood products through needles, syringes, and drug use paraphernalia);
2. sexual transmission (between sexually active drug abusers and also from them to their non-using sexual partners);
3. weakening of the immune system by alcohol and drug use;
4. disinhibition (high risk of unsafe sex or needle use when "high"); and
5. perinatal transmission.

Intravenous drug users are seen as a potential bridge for the AIDS epidemic to move from current high-risk groups to the heterosexual adult population, a fear that has been bolstered by study of the startlingly high number and proportion of sexual partners they have who are not intravenous drug users (Murphy, 1987). For these reasons recent reports have emphasized the need to develop AIDS prevention activities with intravenous drug users (Turner, Miller, & Moses, 1989; Watkins et al., 1988).

USE OF A CONCEPTUAL OVERVIEW

Conceptual models provide useful patterns for designing AIDS prevention campaigns for IV drug abusers. The health belief model (Rosenstock, 1974) may be helpful, because it attends to the beliefs of groups at risk, and differentiates between such aspects as a person's knowledge of the disease, perceived risk of acquiring it, belief in health care guidelines, belief in one's own ability to adhere to the guidelines, and the social support that the person has for adhering to prevention guidelines. Job (1988) has pointed out that in health promotion campaigns the use of fear is often ineffective, contributing to desensitization against the threat, which may be particularly important in attempts to prevent HIV infection.

In San Francisco, AIDS prevention campaigns for drug abusers, sponsored by the San Francisco AIDS Foundation, have followed a course that fits well with the principles of the health belief model. In Spring 1986 the foundation put up the first publicly visible message to drug users, with posters and billboards that stated "DON'T SHARE" (Figure 1). This took place in a time when drug users were not yet generally aware of the dangers of AIDS for them. The DON'T SHARE campaign may have helped to increase awareness and fear of AIDS. The DON'T SHARE message, however, told drug users what *not* to do. In 1987 the AIDS Foundation published its second effort, an "adults only" comic book called THE WORKS: DRUGS, SEX, AND AIDS (Pappas & Dangle, 1987), which spoke in the language of drug users (even to the extent of referring on the cover to "the works" not as hamburger trimmings but rather to a syringe and needle (Figure 2). The comic book provided detailed instructions on preventive activities that drug users could employ, including how to clean needles with bleach and how to use condoms. A third effort came in 1988 with the foundation's BLEACHMAN campaign (Figure 3), which focused on changing social norms. A person in the costume of the 8-feet tall new superhero attended various community functions, media events, and drug treatment programs, demonstrating how to clean needles, giving people a chance to have their picture taken with him, and even handing out BLEACHMAN tee shirts. The BLEACHMAN campaign seemed to attack the social norms of the drug user: Rather than emphasizing knowledge, fear, or living safely, BLEACHMAN worked among drug users because of his outrageousness.

Health education models do not fit perfectly with the medical aspects of AIDS. There is a latency between infection and development of symptomatology, which makes prevention more difficult. Because of a slow progression from infection to disease, by the time the first cases appear in a community, the virus will have established a strong toehold (Moss, 1986). Unfortunately, until some cases appear in their neighborhood it is unlikely that drug abusers will view becoming HIV-infected as a likely event. They may view these prevention messages as simply another intrusion from "straight" (not drug-using) professionals. Similarly, teaching drug users specific behaviors that will prevent HIV infection is unlikely

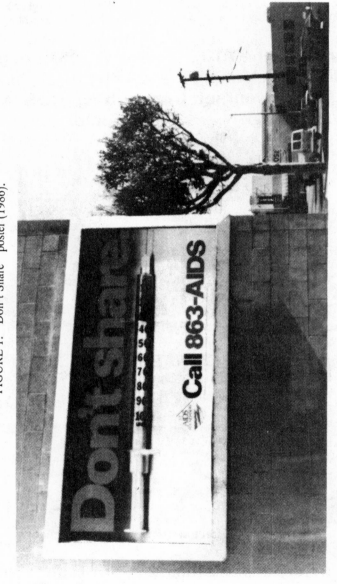

FIGURE 1. "Don't Share" poster (1986).

FIGURE 2. Needle-cleaning Instructions in "The Works" Comic Book (1987). *Note.* Copyright 1987 by the San Francisco AIDS Foundation. Reprinted by permission.

Bleach kills the AIDS virus that gets into used needles. By cleaning them with bleach you will help protect yourself from getting AIDS, and it will not damage the needle.

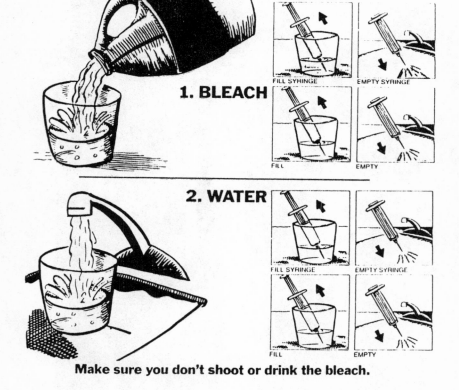

1. BLEACH

FILL SYRINGE EMPTY SYRINGE
FILL EMPTY

2. WATER

FILL SYRINGE EMPTY SYRINGE
FILL EMPTY

Make sure you don't shoot or drink the bleach.

For more facts about AIDS and cleaning needles:

Call 863-AIDS

FIGURE 3. "Bleach Man" character (1988). *Note*. Photograph by Jen Ham. Reprinted by permission.

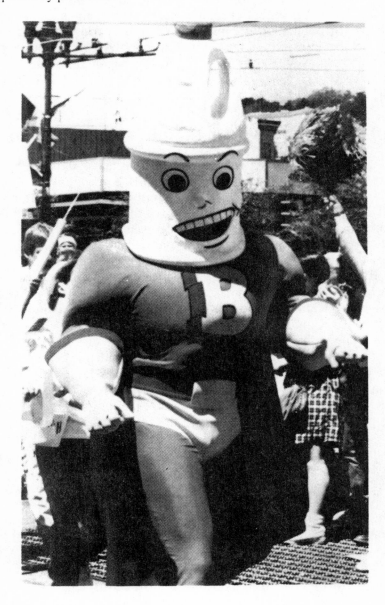

to offer immediate relief of anxiety, because of the latency between infection and testing seropositive. For these reasons it would be unwise to simply import health education campaigns from other diseases or population groups. Instead, prevention programs will need to take into account the unique aspects of AIDS and the people who are at highest risk for acquiring it. It is encouraging to see that Catania, Kegeles, and Coates (1990) have proposed a risk reduction model that is specific to AIDS.

AIDS PREVENTION RESEARCH WITH DRUG ABUSERS

At San Francisco General Hospital's Substance Abuse Services our "psychoeducational" approach to AIDS prevention evolved from work with the families of drug abusers that began before the AIDS era. Our Community Network project was revealing that family members of addicts reacted enthusiastically to a group education approach (Sorensen & Gibson, 1983; Sorensen, Gibson, Bernal, & Deitch, 1985). The 12-hours of group intervention developed similarly to the work of Carol Anderson and associates with the families of schizophrenics, using a technique that they dubbed "psychoeducation" because it combined educational with psychological interventions (Anderson, Hogarty, & Reiss, 1981). As our own Community Network project was coming to a close and we wrote a book for family members, the AIDS epidemic descended so rapidly that we included a chapter about AIDS for the family of drug addicts (Sorensen & Bernal, 1987).

As AIDS became a threat to patients at the program, we adapted the psychoeducational approach to the specific task of preventing HIV infection among drug abusers in treatment. A project entitled "Stop AIDS" had used a group format to help thousands of gay men in San Francisco grapple with the threat of AIDS (Puckett & Bye, 1987), and their approach provided inspiration for the workshops that we developed. To date we have begun to test three psychoeducational approaches, with an accumulation of very encouraging preliminary results. First, we have developed a six-hour group education protocol that includes a new videotape showing drug abusers with AIDS discussing their situation (Sorensen, Gibson, & Boudreaux, 1988). Evaluation of the group has shown clearly that drug abusers in residential treatment gain knowledge about AIDS and change their attitudes toward risk (Sorensen, Gibson, Heitzmann, Dumontet, & Acampora, 1988) and that those in outpatient heroin detoxification also improve their skills and practice of safer sex and safer needle use (Heitzmann et al., 1989). A briefer, individualized psychoeducational intervention with drug abusers has also been developed and shows encouraging preliminary results with drug abusers in outpatient heroin detoxification (Gibson, Wermuth, Lovelle-Drache, Ham, & Sorensen, 1989); and a similar approach is being evaluated with the nondrug-using sexual partners of drug abusers (Gibson et al., 1989). The preliminary results of these studies give some hope that techniques can be developed to enable drug treatment programs to become centers for the prevention of AIDS.

UNMET NEEDS

Even if preventive programs are completely successful in halting the spread of HIV infection (an unlikely possibility) this country will still be facing an onslaught of AIDS cases that is just now appearing. Already between 61,000 and 398,000 injection drug users are infected with HIV (Hahn, Oronato, Jones, & Dougherty, 1989), with estimates that from 1989 through 1993 there will be between 83,800 and 119,100 new AIDS cases among injection drug users (Sisk, Hatziandreu, & Hughes, 1990, p. 38). In preparation for this influx of cases, health psychologists can conduct research that may help health care professionals to cope with AIDS cases among drug abusers. Similarly, the families of AIDS patients and their social support system will suffer from AIDS. Little is known about the types of stresses that family members or caregivers undergo when coping with AIDS in a loved one. More serious from the point of public policy, little is known about the degree to which intravenous drug users have family resources that may help them during their illness, or whether they will need to be completely dependent on publicly-funded health care institutions as their AIDS progresses. These two areas — caregiver and family stresses and resources — have received little attention, and they will become crucial as the AIDS epidemic progresses.

Health psychologists have valuable understanding of the relationships between behavioral principles and physical illness or health. They understand how to reduce disease risk by modifying health beliefs, attitudes, or behaviors. The area of preventing AIDS among intravenous drug users needs to have active involvement of health psychologists, and it can be an applied laboratory in which health psychologists can apply their knowledge. However, unless health psychologists are willing to join this effort, a "psychologist general" will remain a fantasy, and psychologists will have few recommendations to make about AIDS policy. AIDS prevention interventions will not be based upon behavioral principles, but rather upon political expedience.

REFERENCES

Anderson, C. M., Hogarty, G., & Reiss, D. J. (1981). The psychoeducational treatment of schizophrenia. In M. J. Goldstein (Ed.), *New developments in interventions with families of schizophrenics*. San Francisco: Jossey-Bass, pp. 79-94.

Bakeman, R., McCray, E., Lumb, J. R., Jackson, R. E., & Whitley, P. N. (1987). The incidence of AIDS among blacks and hispanics. *Journal of the National Medical Association, 79*, 921-928.

Catania, J. A., Kegeles, S. M., & Coates, T. J. (In press). Towards an understanding of risk behavior: An AIDS risk reduction model. *Health Education Quarterly*.

CDC. (1988, December 26). *AIDS Weekly surveillance Report*. Atlanta, GA: AIDS Program, Center for Infectious Diseases, p. 3.

Faltz. B. G., & Madover, S. (1987). Treatment of substance abuse in patients with HIV infection. *Advances in Alcohol and Substance Abuse, 7*, 143-157.

Gibson, D. R., Wermuth, L., Lovelle-Drache, J., Ham, J., & Sorensen, J. L. (1989). Brief counseling to reduce AIDS risk in intravenous drug users and their sexual partners: Preliminary results. *Counselling Psychology Quarterly*.

Hahn, R. A., Oronato, I. M. Jones, T. S., & Dougherty, J. (1989). Prevalence of HIV infection among intravenous drug users in the United States. *JAMA, 261*, 2677-2684.

Heitzmann, C., A., Sorensen, J. L., Gibson, D. R., Morales, E. R., Costantini, M., Baer, S., & Purnell, S. (1989, April). *AIDS prevention among IV drug abusers: Behavioral changes*. Presented at the meeting of the Society of Behavioral Medicine, San Francisco, CA.

Job, R. F. S. (1988). Effective and ineffective use of fear in health promotion campaigns. *American Journal of Public Health, 78*, 163-167.

Moss, A. M. (1986, April). *AIDS in IV drug users*. Paper presented at the New

Jersey State Health Department meeting on AIDS in the IV drug using community, Newark, NJ.

Murphy, D. L. (1987). Heterosexual contacts of intravenous drug abusers: Implications for the next spread of the AIDS epidemic. *Advances in Alcohol and Substance Abuse*, 7, 89-97.

Pappas, L., (Ed.), & Dangle, L. (Art Dir.). (1987). *The works: Drugs, sex & AIDS* (comic book). San Francisco: San Francisco AIDS Foundation.

Puckett, S. B., & Bye, L. (1987). *The Stop AIDS project: An interpersonal AIDS-prevention program*. San Francisco: The Stop AIDS Project, Inc.

Rosenstock, I. M. (1974). The health belief model in preventive health behavior. *Health Education Monographs*, 2, 355-385.

Sisk, J. E., Hatziandreu, E. J., & Hughes, R. (1990). *The effectiveness of drug abuse treatment: Implications for controlling AIDS/HIV infection*. Washington, DC: Congress of the United States Office of Technology Assessment.

Sorensen, J. L., & Bernal, G. (1987). *A family like yours: Breaking the patterns of drug abuse*. San Francisco: Harper & Row, 1987.

Sorensen, J. L., & Gibson, D. R. (1983). Community network approach to drug abuse treatment. *Bulletin of the Society of Psychologists in Addictive Behaviors*, 2, 99-102.

Sorensen, J. L., Gibson, D., Bernal, G., & Deitch, D. (1985). Methadone applicant dropouts: Impact of requiring involvement of friends or family in treatment. *International Journal of the Addictions*, 20, 1273-1280.

Sorensen, J. L., Gibson, D. R. (executive producers), & Boudreaux, R. (producer/director). (1988). *Conversations about AIDS and drug abuse* (videotape). San Francisco: University of California, San Francisco.

Sorensen, J. L., Gibson, D. R., Heitzmann, C., Dumontet, R., & Acampora, A. (1988). AIDS prevention with drug abusers in residential treatment: Preliminary results. (abstract) *Pharmacology, Biochemistry, & Behavior*, 30, 1988, 548-549.

Turner, C. F., Miller, H. G., & Moses, L. E. (Eds.). (1989). *AIDS: Sexual behavior and intravenous drug use*. Washington, DC: National Academy of Sciences.

Watkins, J. D., Conway-Welch, C., Creedon, J. J., Crenshaw, T. L., DeVos, R. M., Gebbie, K. M., Lee, B. J. III, Lilly, F., O'Connor, J. C., Primm, B. J., Pullen, P. Ser Vaas, C., & Walsh, W. B. (1988). Interim report of the Presidential Commission on the Human Immunodeficiency Virus Epidemic: Chairman's recommendations—Part I. *Journal of Acquired Immune Deficiency Syndrome*, 1, 69-103.